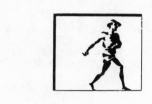

The Complete Book of Birth

From Grantly Dick-Read to Leboyer—a guide for expectant parents to all methods of birth

MORTON WALKER, D.P.M.
BERNICE YOFFE, R.N.
PARKE H. GRAY, M.D.

Illustrations by Tarcisio (Ted) Ciancio

SIMON AND SCHUSTER

NEW YORK

Designed by Stanley S. Drate
Manufactured in the United States of America

2 3 4 5 6 7 8 9 10

Library of Congress Cataloging in Publication Data

Walker, Morton.
   The whole birth book.

   Bibliography: p.
   Includes index.
   1. Pregnancy. 2. Childbirth. 3. Maternal
health services—United States. I. Yoffe, Bernice,
joint author. II. Gray, Parke H., joint author.
III. Title. [DNLM: 1. Labor—Popular works.
2. Delivery—Popular works. 3. Natural childbirth—Methods—Popular works. WQ150.3 W182w]
RG525.W25   618.2   78-26892
ISBN   0-671-24000-5

To Jules Louis Walker,
my prepared childbirth baby,
whom I coached into this world.
—Morton Walker, D.P.M.

To my mother, Florence Hotz, and to all mothers,
who may benefit from this book.
—Bernice Yoffe, R.N.

To my patients, who taught
me what I know in modern obstetrics.
—Parke H. Gray, M.D.

Contents

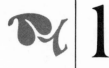 **1**

How Do You Plan to Have the Baby?

When the first baby laughed for the first time,
the laugh broke into a thousand pieces and they
all went skipping about, and that was the
beginning of fairies.
—J. M. BARRIE

We Were Going to Have a Baby

She was sitting on the doctor's table, bare legs dangling out of the white smock. The obstetrician finished examining her and, grinning, said, "Congratulations, Mrs. Walker, you have a fine pregnancy under way."

A baby, that's what we wanted. We felt joyful. I walked around feeling ten feet tall. Inspired! Joan and I kept our secret until the end of the third month.

When our good news became generally known, our family and friends expressed genuine excitement for us. One subject mentioned frequently was the method for giving birth. "How do you plan to have the baby?" became a common question. At first we thought it was a joke. "In the hospital, asleep like everybody else," Joan said. I agreed. But we discovered that was not how childbirth was performed nowadays. Methods for bearing children were changing. There were several available, and almost any of them could be used in our local hospital. We could go to a childbearing unit at a family center. We could even have our baby at home. Joan did not have to go to sleep at all. We had a choice—a whole birth catalog of techniques. A couple of them were more popular among our acquaintances, and different types were in vogue in other parts of the country. We decided to learn about all the procedures for bringing our baby into the world.

Joan and I selected a particular technique for childbearing that seemed most favored locally. We modified it somewhat by adding the best measures taken from a few other techniques. Joan's obstetrician knew them all and helped us choose. I then joined my wife at lectures and demonstrations to learn how to make labor and delivery easier. Luckily we met an instructor who gave prepared childbirth classes in her home, and we attended the classes together.

Joan's having a baby was to be a cooperative effort for us. I became directly involved in the birth of our child. It was a peak experience!

The Main Forms of Childbirth

There are two main forms of childbirth: *participating* and *nonparticipating*. In nonparticipating childbirth, the procedure in common use since Queen Victoria of England popularized chloroform anesthetic delivery, you are in labor, a natural occurrence, but not necessarily helping to push out the baby. Your muscles are not relaxed and don't stay in control of contractions. Sometimes the obstetrician or family physician uses instruments in order to remove your infant from the birth canal. You are sedated during labor and may go to sleep upon delivery. Statistically, more women, at this time, give birth by the well-established, nonparticipating method, but a growing number of mothers-to-be are turning their attention to alternative ways of delivering their babies.

Participating childbirth, or "natural" childbirth, goes back to the time before anesthesia was introduced into obstetrics. This was the only way that women had babies. In primitive cultures it still is the only way—birth in the fields, so to speak—the unaided bearing of a child.

Using the "natural" way, a woman just relaxes and allows the uterus to contract effectively. Nature merely takes its course and the mother follows her instincts. This natural procedure is the way most animals bring forth their young.

There is now a third method of childbirth—the "prepared" method. "Prepared" childbirth differs from "natural" childbirth in that both the mother and father educate themselves in the childbearing process, usually by attending classes, lectures, and demonstrations together. Several weeks or months before the birth itself, you learn techniques to let the pelvic muscles go limp, thus offering less resistance to the baby coming through the birth canal. Through hours of practice you condition yourself to control a contraction and help it to push out the infant.

Besides special relaxation techniques, breathing exercises to accommodate yourself in different *stages* of labor are taught. You become prepared, with the help of the doctor and nurses and your mate, to give birth to your baby without anesthesia and, in most cases, without pain.

Childbirth is a natural experience. It is demanding but not necessarily painful, say the millions of women who have utilized various techniques of prepared childbirth. Labor is exceedingly hard work. But doctors declare, and many mothers confirm, that pain occurs only when you tense up and work *against* nature, instead of with it.

Derivation of the Prepared Methods

As more women prepare for participating childbirth and more obstetricians encourage its practice, the techniques and variations will become more popular around the country. Today, about 40 percent of newborns are delivered this way, and hopefully the number will continue to increase.

The several techniques of prepared childbirth are derived from the time when British obstetrician Grantly Dick-Read first began to practice his particular version of natural childbirth, about 1914. Dr. Dick-Read taught that bearing children is not necessarily painful, that pain comes only because of fear, which may interfere with contractions of uterine muscles that open the womb and push the child out through the birth canal. In his first book, *Natural Childbirth*, published in England in 1933, and later retitled *Childbirth Without Fear*, the obstetrician wrote that pain was psychologically oriented and a consequence of centuries of biblical misrepresentation. He proved through the development of techniques to eliminate fear and reduce muscular tension that a woman in labor can confront her discomfort and deliver a very healthy baby without the use of drugs of any kind.[1]

Dr. Dick-Read was the pioneer in prepared childbirth. He replaced the term "uterine pain" with "uterine contraction." He went out on a limb and advocated the presence of the father in the delivery room. Various exercises were included in his techniques. One of the most successful involved panting during labor contractions to relax skeletal, vaginal, and perineal muscles. Whenever he could, Dr. Dick-Read discouraged the use of analgesic drugs.

The then new British concepts of childbirth found their way to Soviet Russia where Pavlovian psychologists took Dick-Read's idea one step further. They attempted to overcome a woman's fear and pain by conditioning her long before the onset of labor. During the 1940s, Soviet physicians began educating pregnant women to be unafraid of childbirth, and by 1951 hospitals in Moscow, Kharkov, and Leningrad all used the natural- or prepared childbirth method.

A Russian neurologist at the clinics for railway workers in Dnepropetrovsk, Professor Pavol, argued against the use of drugs or hypnosis or suggestion to minimize birth pains. Rather, he advocated making every effort to destroy the false concepts that breed this pain. Then the professor spearheaded efforts to bring universal acceptance of painless childbirth through the psychoprophylactic method. The word *psychoprophylaxis* may be defined as "mind prevention," implying the prevention of pain. Professor Pavol was partially successful. The general application of the method was enforced by a decree from the Soviet Ministry of Health, and Russian women were given an intense physical and psychological education about childbirth during the last months of their pregnancies.

The Psychoprophylactic Method of Childbirth was introduced at a gynecological conference in Paris in 1952 where the French obstetrician Fernand Lamaze first observed it. He then made a trip to Russia to study the technique further. Dr. Lamaze modified the Russian method. He added a rapid, accelerated, chest-breathing technique to prepare his patients for the time when their abdominal muscles would help to expel the baby from the uterus. Dr. Lamaze established a very successful program in France known as "childbirth without pain." This is the birth procedure most widely supported by physicians in the United States and Canada as well as in other countries. It makes use of the work of the Russian scientist Ivan Pavlov, who researched achieving pain relief by conditional reflex.[2]

The Lamaze method concentrates on preventing or lessening pain by psychological and physical means. This includes *effleurage*, a simple massage of the lower abdomen that serves to lessen muscular tension during contractions. The Lamaze method does not make use of analgesics or other drugs, but does not forbid them either. Using the Lamaze techniques, a woman is able to relax while participating actively in labor. She sometimes has by her side a "monitrice," an assistant who usually has been her instructor in the exercise and relaxation techniques.

The methods of Dr. Dick-Read and Dr. Lamaze have been the cornerstones for other procedures. These include Dr. Robert Bradley's *husband coaching*, Dr. Frederick Leboyer's *birth without violence*, the *six steps* of Elisabeth Bing, the unique *decompression bubble*, and others. Yoga or hypnosis can be employed. You may choose the place and period of confinement. For example, in family-centered maternity care, you are hospitalized just for the labor and delivery and nothing more. Then you may go home.

Alternatively, giving birth at home keeps you out of the hospital altogether. A return to home birth is growing in popularity. Unlike bygone days, the father now actively participates in the birth of his baby, with or without the assistance of a lay midwife.

Our reference here is not to the clinic-trained nurse-midwife, whose professional services are being sought more and more. Many nurse-midwives will not deliver babies at home. Others insist that they provide support and care for women who cannot afford good medical attention provided by obstetricians. Therefore, they do deliver midwifery services in the couple's bedroom, using the father as an assistant.

Why Has Participating Childbirth Become So Popular?

There seems to be two reasons in particular for the upsurge by women in their desire to participate in childbirth. First, a great medical revolution has taken place in the area of obstetrics. From a time that goes back about a century when childbirth was a grim, frightening, and unsafe experience for the potential mother, modern medicine has now made it a happy, cheerful, and invulnerable event. Generally, the woman in labor is kept safe and secure. The vast majority of babies are born healthy. Heretofore, pain has been controlled with analgesics, but that practice is being replaced by psychological conditioning of the mother. She is taught to have confidence in her own abilities and in the person assisting her during that important time.

Second, an awakening for women's rights has turned its attention to childbirth as the most feminine of acts. The ability to give birth and how you do it are more symbolic now. In their book, *Our Bodies, Ourselves*, the Boston Women's Health Book Collective wrote:

> There are many steps we can take to become more active, conscious and critical participants in our childbearing experience. We must learn all we can about pregnancy, childbirth and care of ourselves and our children after birth. With this knowledge we can make certain choices. Too often in a critical situation we're not aware of the choices we have. With this knowledge we can sometimes prevent certain complications from arising. We must work on, and along with, doctors and nurses to demystify and deprofessionalize medicine, and persuade them to share their information with us so that we can mutually decide what steps to take if problems arise. . . .

We stress again that it is a strength to be active, to question and criticize procedures; that we have certain rights as patients; and that we need constant support from our husband or friend if we're faced with an important decision while in the midst of labor contractions. . . .

We want to re-own our childbearing experience.[3]

Why Choose Prepared Childbirth

The basic feeling expressed by the couples who choose to prepare for childbirth is that it motivates them to become interested in their own and their infant's health. In the classes you and your mate learn about good nutrition, the need for regular exercise, how to have better posture, and improvements in your whole general being. You practice various breathing and exercise techniques, hear lectures, see films, carry on discussions, and have your questions answered in company with other couples.

In her book, *Having a Baby Can Be a Scream,* comedienne Joan Rivers described the scene:

> It was terrific. They used to put all of us pregnant mommies into gym suits and lay us down on the gym floor to do our exercises. We looked like a relief map of the Rocky Mountains. They explained everything that would happen during labor. At the end, they even showed a movie of a woman giving birth to her baby. I enjoyed that part the most. But for some reason, they threw me out of class. Maybe it was because I asked them to run the movie backward. "Come on, nurse," I shouted, "now let's see the baby disappear."

One of the most important motivations for considering prepared childbirth is the newborn itself. Through practical information and demonstrations about what is happening inside you, you will come to grips with the tasks of pregnancy, labor, and delivery, confinement after delivery, and your relationship with the new baby. You and your mate learn about "parenting." This knowledge and preparation will have a total salutary effect on the infant. Your baby profits!

Sister Mary Charitas, a small, peppery nun who used to teach nursing at St. Louis University School of Nursing and Health Services, summed it up when she described the advantages infants have if their mothers were prepared for childbirth. "The babies are born happier. . . . They're easier to take care of, they're more alert—probably because the mother has not had medication that would make them sleepy,"[4] she said.

Sister Charitas's observations about medications are based on sound medical theory. Obstetricians are aware that an overdependence on anesthetics and other drugs can lead to fetal damage.

If you are motivated to seek this fully participating form of childbearing that eliminates the use of drugs where not absolutely needed, we recommend that you contact The International Childbirth Education Association, Inc., P.O. Box 20852, Milwaukee, Wisconsin 53220. ICEA supports no individual method of preparation but teaches many of the various modern approaches to childbirth. Formed in 1960, this international education association has local chapters throughout the United States and Canada. Probably there is a chapter near you.

Times and Practices Have Changed

Times have changed and women have more options. Practices in childbirth have altered exceedingly. Doctors and nurses are informed and in most cases are considerate of patients' needs and desires. Hospitals are spotlessly antiseptic. Mothers and fathers are becoming highly educated about the birth process, and fathers frequently take on the role of obstetrical assistant or coach to his mate. Birth has become a joyful, cooperative effort dedicated to bringing forth a happy and healthy baby.

The only requirement for a father to be allowed into the labor and delivery rooms is that the couple attend preparation-for-childbirth classes together. Six to eight weeks of class attendance given one evening a week by a childbirth educator, who often is a registered nurse, teaches the couple the goals and means of prepared childbirth. Father and mother become mentally ready for him to wheel her right into the labor room. Then they use what they have learned.

Yes, there is discomfort from the contractions—no denying that—and each new one grows stronger. But the mother remains in control of her labor just as their instructor has promised. It is childbirth without suffering. Lots of smiles. A boosted morale for the woman about to give birth. Teamwork between lovers soon to be parents. The man is there to offer concern, support, understanding, and esteem. His strength is infectious and gives her strength and confidence. A chemistry flows between them. His eyes peeping out from behind the surgical mask let her know he loves her. With her hand holding his, she pushes on cue to cause the baby's head to crown. The doctor and nursing staff cheer her on. It is one big happening! It's very special!

NOTES FOR CHAPTER ONE

1. Grantly Dick-Read, *Childbirth Without Fear* (New York: Harper & Row, 1952).

2. Lou Joseph, *A Doctor Discusses Natural Childbirth* (Chicago: Budlong Press, 1977).

3. The Boston Women's Health Book Collective, *Our Bodies, Ourselves* (New York: Simon and Schuster, 1976).

4. "Obstetrics, Fewer Drugs for Happier Mothers," *Time*, September 25, 1964.

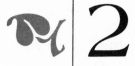

2

Preparation for Pregnancy

The family you come from isn't as important
as the family you're going to have.
—RING LARDNER

You Determine Your Child's Destiny

Some personalities in history—Goethe was one of them—were convinced that the constellation under which a person is born has a great influence on his or her destiny. This line of thinking naturally suggests that the birth of a baby should be fixed in accordance with favorable constellations in the heavens. But in our "practical" society the decision of when to have a baby usually comes from more down-to-earth factors.

The things that really influence a child's destiny may be whether or not the house is spacious enough, whether the income is large enough, whether there is sufficient time to spare, or other tangible conditions. The emotional need for parenthood also plays a very large role in the decision to conceive or not. Because of the major advances in and use of contraception, pregnancy usually becomes an active choice of most couples. And if pregnancy does occur by accident, a legal abortion can end it.

Most often childbearing is, and should be, a choice made on earth and not in heaven. The position of the stars and any other obscure influences should not be involved. You determine your child's destiny. Preparing for pregnancy and being physically, mentally, and emotionally fit will give the baby a head start at being a winner in life.

The Best Possible Health Before Pregnancy

Both partners should have a positive outlook when making the conscious decision to become parents. Hopefully your decision arises out of love, and you have thought this through thoroughly and intelligently. Of course, it is most important for the woman to be physically fit, but the father-to-be should also try to stay in good condition. He can assist his mate in any nutrition, exercise, or weight control program that may need to be followed.[1]

During pregnancy, your body will be changing rapidly. Nine months is too short a time to get yourself in perfect physical condition. If you have not maintained your ideal weight before the pregnancy, you won't be able to achieve it during the pregnancy, since it will be deleterious to the fetus actually to diet. Or if you have weakened abdominal muscles, you may not adequately be able to perform the sit-ups which will strengthen those muscles needed to push out the baby. To build stamina, jogging is excellent, but during the pregnancy you might not be able to jog the daily mile or two required unless you start your jogging program before the nine months begins. Women who incorporate yoga into their pregnancy, labor, and delivery have probably been practicing the yoga disciplines for months or years before. It is quite difficult to take on yoga while you're pregnant and have it be 100 percent effective.

We emphasize that you should attempt to be in the best possible health when you conceive and remain that way throughout the entire pregnancy. Since you will not know the exact time that conception occurs, you ought to begin preparing yourself a year before then. Eliminate smoking and the taking of drugs. Stop drinking. Exercise regularly. Get yourself into the best possible physical condition. This chapter suggests how to proceed.

Prepregnancy and Prenatal Nutrition

Good nutrition before conception will eliminate a lot of the complaints women have when they become pregnant.

On the second visit to their physicians it is not unusual for some women to say, "Gee, Doctor, I'm so tired all the time. I'm constipated, too!" Inadequate nutrition prior to pregnancy is often the cause of many of the problems during the early prenatal time. By getting the proper nourishment through a good diet before conception, you will be able to avoid these problems.

There are general rules to follow for prepregnancy and prenatal nutrition, as well as for nutrition practices throughout the rest of your life. Use the following suggestions as a guide:

- Try to include all the basic foods in your diet. They include milk and other dairy products, bread, vegetables, fruits, meat, poultry, and fish.
- Avoid artificial colorings, flavorings, and other chemical additives in your basic foods.
- Use whole-meal flour of the various grains, such as wheat, oats, rye, and others whenever possible. Eliminate white flour when you can.
- Use mostly vegetable fats such as sunflower seed oil, safflower seed oil and linoleate oil which are cold-pressed and in a natural state. And don't use much of any fats and oils.
- Limit drinks containing caffeine, sugar, or saccharin.
- Where possible, serve and eat natural, unprocessed foods.

The Four Basic Daily Food Groups

The best nutrition for prepregnancy and the prenatal period will be supplied by making sure you eat full measures daily in the four basic food groups. These will include four or more servings of enriched or whole-grain *breads and cereals*; four or more servings of dark green or yellow *vegetables*, citrus fruits and other *fruits; protein* consisting of meats, fish, poultry, eggs, or cheese, with dry beans, peas or nuts as alternates; *milk products*. This combination of foods is the foundation for a nutritious diet. Use more of the basics and other foods as needed for growth, for activity, and for desirable weight.

The menu plan we recommend for minimum amounts of food from each of the four basic groups is shown in Table 1. Following this menu plan will allow you a means of including the four important food groups in one day's meals.

General Advice About Wholesome Living

A lot of people enjoy a sweet after dinner, but we have taken a stand against daily use of refined carbohydrates as desserts if you are preparing to have a baby. Whipped cream, ice cream, cookies, candy bars, and various pastries should be eliminated. Fill in for them with a naturally sweet dessert like crisp apples, plump raisins, ripe bananas, fresh oranges, and other fruits.

TABLE 1
THE DAILY MENU PLAN FOR PREPREGNANCY
AND PRENATAL NUTRITION

BREAKFAST

citrus fruit or melon

hot or cold, nonsugared cereal or egg or both

whole-wheat toast or roll*

skimmed milk or herb tea†

DINNER

fish, lean meat, or poultry

green or other vegetables, steamed or raw

sprouted bread or muffin*

skimmed milk or herb tea†

fresh fruit or nuts for dessert‡

LUNCH OR SUPPER

fish, lean meat, or poultry

seven-grain bread*

green or yellow vegetable

skimmed milk or herb tea†

fresh fruit in season‡

Vary your menus to suit your taste.

In the protein group, you should have as much protein as four ounces cooked lean meat ($\frac{1}{3}$ pound raw). About equal amounts of protein come from . . .

two ounces (57 grams) cooked lean meat, poultry, or fish

two eggs

two slices cheese, American or Swiss (two ounces or 57 grams)

four rounded tablespoons cottage cheese (four ounces or 114 grams)

four tablespoons peanut butter (two ounces or 57 grams)

one cup cooked dried beans or peas

$1\frac{1}{2}$ cup milk

An average serving of vegetables or fruits is $\frac{1}{2}$ cup; of bread is one slice; of cereal is $\frac{1}{2}$ to $\frac{3}{4}$ cup.

* Avoid eating bread, rolls or muffins made with white flour.

† Avoid coffee and cola drinks, which the Food and Drug Administration warned recently may cause birth defects.

‡ Avoid any form of dessert made with sugar and/or white flour.

Note: The nutritional statements made here have been reviewed by the Council on Foods and Nutrition of the American Medical Association and found consistent with current authoritative medical opinion.

While there is no objective evidence that caffeine in tea, coffee, and cola drinks is directly harmful to the mother or infant, we believe it is a good idea to cut down on these beverages as well. Many of the symptoms of nervousness or rapid heartbeats among women can possibly be traced directly to consumption of caffeine. Coffee drinking often becomes compulsive—start with one cup and usually it leads in time to drinking a dozen a day.

You can point an accusing finger at alcohol in the same way. "I'll just have one cocktail to relax before my husband comes home," a woman may say. But one leads to another drink when he comes in—then another with dinner. Drinking as a routine sneaks up on you until it is difficult to break the habit.

The drinking of alcohol by pregnant women has been shown without question to be injurious to fetal growth. Medical studies indicate that drinking more than four ounces of alcohol daily—in the form of whiskey, wine, or beer—considered an excess—will cause *fetal alcohol syndrome*. This condition leaves a newborn with improper development of the brain. The baby will be born with an undersized head.

Smaller amounts of alcohol have been shown to be less destructive so that an occasional cocktail or glass of wine probably is not harmful. But if you drink cocktails every day, you will be exposing your baby to low levels of alcohol throughout its fetal development.

A small amount of drinking daily may not build a true physiological addiction, but psychological addiction is quite possible and quite common. For this reason we believe you should sharply limit your drinking during the prepregnancy and prenatal periods.

Smoking: The Great Destroyer

Smoking deserves a discussion by itself. If you smoke while pregnant, nicotine from the burning tobacco will cause constriction of your blood vessels, thereby reducing the blood flow to the uterus. Your fetus will receive an inadequate amount of nourishment as a result. By smoking only ten cigarettes a day you stand a significantly greater chance of losing your baby, either before it is born or in the first four weeks of infancy, than a nonsmoking mother.

If your child survives, he or she will have a much greater chance, in the early school years, of being behind those children, in reading ability and social adjustment, whose mothers did not smoke during pregnancy. These are proven medical and sociological facts. Not theory! They come from a report by the Surgeon General of the United States (*The Health Consequences of Smoking—A Report of the Surgeon General: 1971*).

Another report (*Smoking and Health Now—A Report of the Royal College of Physicians*) backs up the U.S. report. Both reports are based on a worldwide survey of continuing medical research.

Studies were independently pursued in nine separate countries. All arrived at the same stark conclusion: Nicotine or some other agent in cigarette smoke besets the fetus with potentially disastrous consequences.

Carbon monoxide may be the offending substance. This gas of burning tobacco present in the blood of the smoking mother may work its way into the baby's circulation. The most apparent effect is to retard the growth of the unborn child.

The studies further show that if you smoke during the prenatal time you are more likely to produce a baby of lower birth weight. The more you smoke, the more you increase such risk. Babies of smoking mothers average approximately half a pound less than that of babies born to nonsmoking mothers. Sometimes this one-half pound can be the crucial difference in a newborn infant's fight for life.

"A premature baby will most likely be smaller throughout its life," said Henry L. Harris, M.D., who is instructor in pediatrics at the Albert Einstein College of Medicine of Yeshiva University, Bronx, New York. "It will be less well developed, less muscular than his contemporaries. We are not fully able to measure the subtle changes that occur, but medical science can project that a seven-and-a-half-pound baby who should have been born eight pounds probably would have been better in sports or even more intelligent, if it had developed in the womb to its full potential."

More than fifteen medical studies have zeroed in on the destructive effects of smoking on the health of a child born of a smoking mother. We will cite just three, as examples.

A study of two thousand pregnancies conducted in Sheffield, England, uncovered that almost 8 percent of women who smoked lost their babies, compared with only 4 percent of those who did not smoke. The researchers, in extrapolating their findings, projected that one in five of the smoking mothers who lost their babies would probably have had a successful pregnancy if she had quit smoking at the onset of pregnancy or before.

A similar finding was found in the laboratory among pregnant rhesus monkeys. Two years of tests were carried out. The tests showed that nicotine introduced into the monkey mother's bloodstream increased acidity in the fetus, impaired its heart rate, blood pressure, and oxygen supply.

Finally, Professor Neville R. Butler, director of Bristol University's child-health department, in a study called *Britain's National Birthday Trust Perinatal Mortality Survey,* discovered that babies born of smoking mothers suffer distinct long-term disabilities. During the week of March 3, 1958, newborns in England, Scotland, and Wales were tested. Then, in 1965, when the children were seven years old, they were retested thoroughly for school performance and physical well-being.

Professor Butler was able to draw a very clear profile of these children. The results were disheartening both to the parents and the test authorities. Each seven-year-old whose mother had smoked heavily during and after her fourth month of pregnancy was a half-inch shorter than children of nonsmoking mothers. The child was also four months behind the average reading level for his age. The child was significantly less able to adjust to the school environment, was generally clumsier at handling objects, and had an impaired spatial sense. Such a child born of a smoking mother, in fact, was among the lower 10 percent of his or her class at copying drawings of simple designs.

These unfortunate children were burdened with scholastic handicaps and physical handicaps which were directly attributable to smoking during pregnancy.

Sugar: Sweet Mystery of Life

Many of us have an innate sweet tooth which seems to have been with us since birth. But interestingly sugar can be a disturbing addiction even to the child not yet born. Sugar presents a sweet mystery of life.

It has been observed that if saccharin is injected into the womb, the human fetus will increase its swallowing of the sweetened amniotic fluid.

Newborn rats given a choice will consume sugar water in preference to a nutritious diet, even to the point of malnutrition and death.

Our analysis reveals that you should avoid sugar consumption during your preparation for pregnancy and childbirth. In January 1977, the Senate Select Committee on Nutrition and Human Needs urged Americans to reduce their sugar consumption by 40 percent. Cited for such evils as drawing away the attention of youngsters from more nutritious foodstuffs, enhancing obesity, ruining teeth, and causing heart disease and diabetes, sugar has proven to be the most injurious of the main components of the American diet.

A young, healthy woman who was five foot two inches tall, a bit pudgy but not strikingly fat, in her sixth month of pregnancy was discovered to have overt diabetes. She had an elevated blood sugar and was spilling sugar in her urine. In carefully going into her dietary history, we learned that she was eating quantities of sweets each day in the form of soft drinks, iced tea, candy, and just adding sugar to everything she consumed. Simply by eliminating her excess sugar intake and putting her on a normal caloric requirement—not even a strict diabetic diet—we were able to see her gestational diabetes disappear completely.

Since 70 percent of the sugar consumed in today's American diet is "hidden" in processed foods, you should check the labels of the packaged soups, cereals, salad dressings, soft drinks, ketchup, sauces, peanut better, dessert mixes, and other items in your pantry. See how many list sugar or corn syrup as a main ingredient. Try to avoid these sugared substances. Better yet, try to avoid processed foods in general.

The body has no physiological need for sucrose (sugar) that cannot be satisfied by other more nutritious foods such as fruits and vegetables. The purported need for sugar as "quick energy" is a myth, except in a few rare situations, such as a diabetic in insulin shock.

Essentially we are saying that no longer is there a sweet mystery to sugar intake. An excess of sugar consumption can lead to potential disease and disability for you and your unborn child.

Misunderstandings About Table Salt Intake

No one should attempt a salt-free diet unless he or she has been specifically directed by an expert. This is especially true if you are expecting a baby. Life cannot be maintained without sufficient salt, and common table salt is the substance most often used to ensure this maintenance. But excessive salt intake *can* cause serious disturbances. Foods that contain high concentrations of sodium, the element that combines with chloride to form table salt, should be avoided. Indeed, there are misunderstandings in general about salt intake.

The body of an average woman, whether or not in the process of creating a new life in her uterus, requires the ingestion of at least ten grams (one-third ounce) of salt daily. It is the habit of Americans to take in about twice this much. And Europeans even more. Vegetarians may possibly need twenty grams of salt daily but not meat eaters.

Sodium chloride tends to drive the mineral potassium out of body cells, and a good way to ensure a good potassium-sodium balance in the body is to cut down on salt intake. If not, signs of potassium depletion can develop. They are: listlessness, fatigue, weakness, constipation, insomnia, slow and irregular heartbeat, absent reflexes, mental confusion, and soft, flabby muscles. Also, neuromuscular and regular muscle functions can be impaired. We therefore recommend that you limit your table salt intake and avoid the foods which are high in sodium listed in Table 2.

We have presented this discussion of proper nutrition as a preparation for pregnancy because what you eat is the most vital and most

TABLE 2
FOODS TO AVOID THAT ARE HIGH IN SODIUM

I. *Meat and Other Protein Foods*

  A. Salted and smoked meats such as:

bacon	ham
bologna	meats koshered by salting
chipped or corned beef	luncheon meats
frankfurters	sausage
smoked tongue	commercial egg substitutes

  B. Salted or smoked fish such as:

caviar	herring
anchovies	sardines, etc.
salted or dried cod	

  C. Processed cheese (unless low-sodium) such as:

Roquefort
Camembert
Gorgonzola

II. *Bread Group*

  A. Any bread or rolls with salt toppings

pretzels	salted crackers
potato chips	popcorn, salted
heavily salted snack food, such as cheese crackers, etc.	

III. *Vegetables*

  A. Anything that is prepared in brine or heavily salted such as:

sauerkraut	olives
relishes	pickles

IV. *Fats*

salted nuts	salt pork
olives	dips
bacon and bacon fat	

V. *Miscellaneous Foods*

meat and steak sauces	garlic salt	meat extracts and
barbecue sauces	onion salt	tenderizers
soy sauce	celery salt	dehydrated soups
Worcestershire sauce	canned soups	prepared mustard
catsup	table salt	prepared horseradish
chili sauce	bouillon cubes	monosodium glutamate (MSG)

controllable factor in your preventing the birth of an unhealthy child or a premature birth. The more successful you are in holding your fetus to full term, the more effective you can be at producing a healthy baby.

Developments in obstetrics in the past few years have been so phenomenal that the future for the newborn is brighter than ever before. In these developments, research pediatricians have been working hand in glove with obstetricians, so close that there has now developed a new medical specialty involving both obstetricians and pediatricians.

One of the professional organizations that represents this new medical specialty on obstetrical management and infant outcome is The American Foundation for Maternal and Child Health, Inc., 30 Beekman Place, New York, New York 10022. It performs interdisciplinary research in maternal and child health whose main focus is on the perinatal period (any of the times immediately before, during, or after birth). The implication for such research is the alteration of various factors in the birth and neonatal history of the child for future mental and physical development. You can acquire more information about enhancing those factors for your own potential infant by contacting the foundation directly.

Good Advice for Pregnancy Nutrition

One in every thirty-five children born in the United States today will eventually be diagnosed as mentally retarded or as having some form of significant neurological handicap. One of every ten children in the United States has been found to have minimal brain dysfunction or a learning disability. These statistics indicate an alarming increase in birth defects in this country closely related to weight control diets, extreme salt restriction, sugar intake, food additives, and use of diuretics (foods that increase urine flow) during pregnancy.

Tom Brewer, M.D., and his wife, Gail, authors of *What Every Pregnant Woman Should Know: The Truth About Diet and Drugs in Pregnancy*,[2] believe that restricting a woman's weight gain during pregnancy leads to smaller babies. They feel that birth weight is the single most important factor in predicting a child's future health and mental development.

The Brewers' advice to expectant mothers:

- Don't be overanxious about weight gain.
- Eat according to appetite, with *good nutrition* as the primary consideration.
- Salt foods to taste but not excessively.
- Avoid unnecessary drugs, particularly diuretics.

The Brewers recently had occasion to practice what they preach. In May 1977, Gail Brewer gave birth to a daughter, Cornelia—nine pounds two ounces and the picture of health.

Essential Nutrients

Table 3 is a summary of essential nutrients you need for a successful pregnancy. A baby born before it is mature enough or big enough to survive can easily die or survive with whatever effects may remain from the fight for survival. To avoid prematurity or a dangerously low birth weight, do not skimp on your nutrition program. The National Research Council Committee on Maternal Nutrition encourages this view. Overly strict weight control during the prenatal period contributes to low birth weight and stillbirth. We, therefore, concur with the American Academy of Husband-Coached Childbirth whose members say: "It is far more important to have a full range of sound nutrition than to limit natural weight gain."[3]

TABLE 3
SUMMARY OF ESSENTIAL NUTRIENTS

Essential Nutrients	Function in the Body	Good Food Sources	Comments
Protein	Required for growth, maintenance, and repair of body tissues. Helps to make hemoglobin, form antibodies to fight infection, and supply energy.	Meat, poultry, fish, eggs, milk, cheese, soybeans, beans, peas, grains, and nuts.	Foods of animal origin contain protein of better nutritional value than foods of plant origin. However, eating plant-origin foods is recommended more.
Carbohydrates (starches, sugars, and celluloses)	Starches and sugars are major sources of energy for internal and external work and to maintain body temperature. Celluloses furnish bulk in diet.	Grains (wheat, oats, corn, rice) and grain products (flour, bread, cereal, macaroni, etc.), sugar, jams and jellies, candy, soft drinks, honey, and most fruits and vegetables.	Excess carbohydrates in diet are converted into fat and are stored in the body. Processed carbohydrates are less desirable than natural carbohydrates. Avoid eating processed carbohydrates, if possible.

SOURCE: Supplied by the courtesy of the American Osteopathic Association, 212 East Ohio Street, Chicago, Illinois 60611. This table has been modified somewhat by the authors.

TABLE 3—*Continued*

Fats	Concentrated source of energy. Carry fat-soluble vitamins and help body to use them. Fats also make up part of cell structure, cushion vital organs; some contain linoleic acid, believed to be essential for health.	Butter, margarine, cooking and salad oils, cream, most cheeses, nuts, bacon, fatty meats, and—to some extent—whole milk, eggs, chocolate, and most meat.	"Unsaturated" fat or linoleic acid found in most vegetable oils; poultry and fish oils have more than animal fats. Avoid eating saturated fats, if possible.
Minerals Calcium	Builds bones and teeth; aids in proper functioning of muscles, heart, and nerves; helps in blood coagulation.	Milk, hard cheese, and in kale, mustard, turnip, and collard greens. Also some in oysters, shrimp, salmon, clams, and in other dairy products.	Calcium is the most abundant mineral in the body. Getting it from vegetable sources is more advantageous.
Iron	One of the constituents of hemoglobin, which carries oxygen to the tissues by blood circulation. Iron is present in all body cells.	All kinds of liver are the best sources of iron; also meat, egg yolk, legumes, molasses, dark green leafy vegetables, peaches, prunes, apricots, raisins, and food made with enriched flour or cereal.	Iron deficiency is most common in growing children, adolescent girls, pregnant or nursing women.
Phosphorus	Builds bones and teeth (with other minerals); important in a number of body systems involving fats, carbohydrates, salts, and enzymes.	Milk, cheese, egg yolk, meat, fish, fowl, legumes, nuts, whole-grain cereals.	Some forms of phosphorus are not utilized if the vitamin D level is inadequate in the diet.
Iodine	Required to regulate the exchange of food for energy.	Iodized salt best protection; also salt-water fish.	The need for iodine is increased in adolescence and during pregnancy.
Potassium	Needed to maintain fluid balance within the cell; regulates muscular and nervous irritability; necessary for regular heart rhythm.	Meat, fish, fowl, cereals, fruits, vegetables.	Deficiency in diet is uncommon, but may occur in connection with some diseases.

TABLE 3—*Continued*

Sodium	Protects body against excessive fluid loss, regulates muscle and nerve irritability, and maintains water balance.	Table salt, meat, fish, fowl, milk, eggs, and sodium compounds.	Excessive salt intake dangerous for persons subject to hypertension and kidney disorders.
Fluorine	In small quantities protects the teeth against cavities. In larger quantities, fluorine causes mottling of the teeth.	Milk, eggs, and fish; many communities add low concentrations of fluorine to drinking water.	Prolonged high intake of fluorine may cause skeletal abnormalities.

Other minerals which are considered essential for good health are chlorine, sulfur, magnesium, manganese, copper, zinc, cobalt, and molybdenum. In most cases, diet provides adequate intake. However, zinc may have to be supplemented.

Vitamin A	Important for skeletal growth and normal tooth structure; necessary for healthy mucous membranes in mouth, nose, throat, digestive and urinary tracts; and essential for night vision.	Fish-liver oils, liver, butter, cream, milk, cheese, egg yolk, dark green and yellow vegetables, yellow fruits, and fortified margarine.	Fat soluble; destroyed by oxidation and very high temperatures.
Vitamin B$_1$ (Thiamine)	Necessary to help convert sugar and starches into energy.	Pork, liver, heart, kidney, milk, yeast, whole-grain and enriched cereals and breads, soybeans, legumes, peanuts, and wheat germ.	Quickly destroyed by heat in neutral or alkaline solutions.
Vitamin B$_2$ (Riboflavin)	Essential link in the body's use of protein, carbohydrates, and fats for energy.	Milk, powdered whey, liver, kidney, heart, meats, eggs, green leafy vegetables, dried yeast.	Decomposes quickly in light or in alkaline solutions.
Vitamin B$_6$ (Pyridoxine, pyridoxal, pyridoxamine)	Important for the body's use of protein, carbohydrates, and fat; aids in formation of hemoglobin.	Wheat germ, meat, liver, kidney, whole-grain cereals, soybeans, peanuts, corn; some in milk and green vegetables.	Water soluble; destroyed by ultraviolet light and heat.

TABLE 3—*Continued*

Vitamin B$_{12}$ (Cobalamin)	Essential for forming red blood cells; helps in forming all cells in body and in functioning of nervous system.	Milk, eggs, cheese, liver, kidney, muscle meats contain small amounts needed for normal body functioning.	Inactivated by air or light; water soluble.
Folic acid	Needed for use of protein in body and for regeneration of blood cells.	Green leafy vegetables, liver, kidney, yeast, and—in lesser quantities—many foods.	Easily inactivated in sunlight and acid solutions.
Pantothenic acid	Necessary for the body's use of carbohydrates, fats, and protein in conjunction with other substances.	Almost universally present in plant and animal tissue. Loss of 50% in milling of flour; 33% lost in cooking meat.	Water soluble; destroyed easily by dry heat and alkaline.
Niacin	Active in normal functioning of tissues, particularly of the skin, gastrointestinal tract, and nervous system; with other vitamins, used in converting carbohydrates to energy.	Lean meat, liver, kidney, whole-grain and enriched cereals and breads, green vegetables, peanuts, yeast.	Water soluble; stable to heat, air, light.
Biotin	Essential for the functioning of many body systems and use of food for energy.	Liver, kidney, molasses, milk, yeast, egg yolk, and green vegetables.	Water soluble; quite stable in heat, air, and light.
Vitamin C (Ascorbic acid)	Essential for the formation of collagen, a protein which supports the body structures; needed for the absorption of iron, some proteins, and folic acid.	Citrus fruits, strawberries, cantaloupe, tomatoes, cabbage, potatoes, green peppers, and broccoli.	Water soluble; destroyed by heat, air, and light, as well as by aging, drying, and copper contact.

TABLE 3—*Continued*

Vitamin D	Promotes normal bone and tooth development; necessary for absorption and stabilization of calcium and phosphorus.	Fish-liver oils, fortified milk, exposure to sunlight; very small amounts in butter, liver, and egg yolks.	Fat soluble; stable to heat and air.
Vitamin E (Tocopherol)	Protects the body's store of vitamin A and the tissue fat from destructive oxidation; also prevents breakdown of red blood corpuscles.	Oils of wheat germ, rice germ, cottonseed, and the germs of other seeds; green leafy vegetables, nuts, and legumes.	Fat soluble; breaks down in presence of lead and iron salts, alkalies, and ultraviolet light.
Vitamin K	Essential for blood clotting.	Green leafy vegetables such as alfalfa, spinach, cabbage; liver.	Fat soluble; unstable to light.
Water	Essential for life; is the solvent for all products of digestion, the medium of body fluids; regulates body temperature.	Beverages, many solid foods (for example, potatoes contain 78% water).	One-half to two-thirds of the body is made up of water.

Physical Fitness Prior to Pregnancy

Pregnancy represents a significant strain on the heart. During pregnancy your total blood volume increases by two pints so that the heart has to work much harder. Your body is expanding with the increased circulation needed for the uterus and placenta. In order best to handle this extra cardiovascular strain, you should prepare yourself ahead of time with a routine of exercises including aerobics, jogging, swimming, bicycle riding, tennis, or any other sports that will make the heart pump the blood around your body faster. By being in good cardiovascular condition, when you become pregnant you will not be bothered by shortness of breath, extreme tiredness, and other common symptoms of poor body conditioning. Your heart muscle will be able to cope with the increased work it faces to provide the additional circulation needed.

Pregnancy also puts an overload on the musculoskeletal system. Changes occur in the bones and joints. The ligaments of the pelvis

become softened and the bones at the pelvic girdle may slip around a little. And, of course, you'll have a bulging belly that will put you off balance slightly and cause swayback. If your muscle tone is poor, you are going to be bothered by backaches, leg cramps, and other pressure symptoms from the growing fetus. Your muscles have to be strong enough to hold everything together. Make it your personal rule to go into training as soon as the thought of becoming pregnant comes to mind. Prepregnancy training is extremely important.

Two exercises to begin a training program in preparation for pregnancy are jogging and swimming. We highly recommend them. They can both be practiced although either one is effective.

A fine prepregnancy swimming program would consist of a continuous one-half-mile swim performed in thirty-five minutes, four times weekly. In the local YWCA pool this means swimming back and forth for thirty-five laps, a common practice among our patients.

One of our patients visited us, saying, "I think I'm in early labor. I have felt contractions all night."

We said, "It is now eleven A.M. Why didn't you call in at nine A.M. when the office opened?"

She said, "At nine o'clock I was over at the Y swimming. I swam a half hour and decided it is time to notify my obstetrician." The physically fit young woman had her baby at four that afternoon.

We should mention that this woman did feel contractions while swimming, but she felt lighter while floating in the water. She had no discomfort. The buoyancy of water seems to relieve the force of each contraction.

Yoga: Excellent for Physical and Mental Fitness

Yoga (Figure 1) is an excellent form of exercise, not only for its physical effect but for the mental relaxation and spiritual uplift it produces as well. Practicing yoga throughout your prenatal period and thereafter will be advantageous. Yoga may also be beneficial during labor and delivery. For more information on the yoga technique for use in childbirth turn to Chapter 11.

If you are new to yoga discipline, you may wonder when is the best time to begin a course of yoga as a preparation for pregnancy. We believe that anytime is a good time. Some yoga teachers suggest it is best to begin during the moon's first quarter, and when your breath flow is through your left nostril. Since we are not experts in this discipline, it would be best for you to consult your prospective yoga teacher.

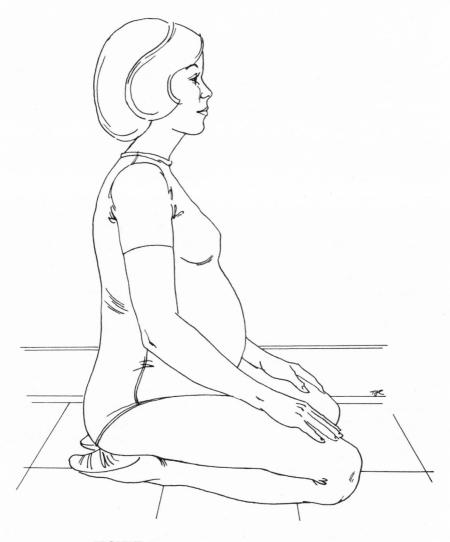

FIGURE 1

Yoga helps to bring mental relaxation. A good mental attitude is very important when preparing to create a new life, and conception will come easier if you maintain mental and physical relaxation.

An important part of yoga's effectiveness is its emphasis on breathing. The discipline's various breathing exercises will bring more oxygen to the cells. A good way to ensure this is to practice outdoors when possible. When your practice is confined indoors, the room must be well-ventilated, cheerful, dry, and free of dust and noise.[4]

A Note on Care of Feet and Legs

During pregnancy posture is extremely important because the body carries additional weight as the fetus develops. The shoes you wear must not only be appropriate but must be fitted with care. Therefore, this is not the time for wearing high heels or a loose, casual flat shoe. The proper shoe is a good, supportive leather or rubber-soled oxford. The upper should be made of leather or a strong fabric, and the heel should be less than an inch and a half in height. Because your feet expand during the day, new shoes should be fitted in the late afternoon or evening when the feet are closer to their maximum length. And since your feet may expand as the weight you carry increases, you might have the new shoes fitted with extra insoles when you buy them. Then you can remove the insoles later to enlarge the shoes.

Give immediate attention to any unusual growths on the feet such as corns, calluses, warts, or ingrown nails. Do not let these pesky annoyances cause you undue pain or fatigue. See a podiatrist about them. If a red, netlike appearance of varicose veins occurs on the legs, wear strong elastic stockings of narrow mesh to support the veins.[5]

Poor Health Habits to Modify for Pregnancy

Some women tend to neglect their teeth, but dental care before and during pregnancy is vital. The gums become more engorged with blood when you are pregnant, and they tend to bleed more. Gums in poor condition can cause discomfort. We recommend that you see your dentist for a thorough prophylaxis as part of a prepregnancy program.

It is surprising how little drinking water most people take in each day. The usual source of body fluid for many Americans comes from cola drinks and other sweetened sodas. That is a terrible habitual practice. Instead, you should seek a definite intake of at least six glasses of purified water daily. And if you suspect the city's water supply is not as pure as standards demand, drink spring water, bottled water, filtered water, or distilled water, but not tap water. Try to avoid drinking heavily chlorinated and fluorinated waters. Studies indicate that chlorinated water causes cancer. Housewives who drank tap water at home, as opposed to women who worked in offices and drank bottled spring water, had a higher incident of bladder cancer because of pollution and perhaps from their city water being chlorinated and fluorinated, according to information published in the osteopathic and chiropractic literature.

We emphasize that you should get seven or eight hours of restful sleep every night. If you tend to have insomnia and cannot relax at night, take a daytime nap as an adjunct.

As a matter of fact, adopting some form of purposeful relaxation or diversion during the day would be a good idea. Some people benefit enormously by incorporating twenty minutes of meditation or mind control into their day's activities. Meditation will separate you from all the usual tensions of living. Take up some quiet hobby. It could be handicrafts such as crocheting, knitting, needlepoint, or sewing. Hook a rug. Build furniture. Make candles. Play music. There are so many new things that are available now for your diversion. Try to make it a manual activity rather than a mental one. This will be the best means of getting out of the poor health habit of confronting daily pressures and tensions and absorbing too much stress.

Psychological Preparation for Pregnancy

We presumed at the beginning of this chapter that you and your mate have thought through the many ramifications of parenthood before going about conceiving a baby. You love each other. Then you came to a mutual, conscious decision to conceive.

The decision to become a parent, however, carries with it the responsibility of learning what parenting is all about. Prior to becoming pregnant, you and your mate will be preparing your bodies physically. At the same time we suggest that you prepare yourselves psychologically.

Many new parents are surprised and some are ill-prepared for the amount of effort that goes into the care of this little infant. You will be taking on an emotional commitment as well as a financial one, and committing hours each day to the baby. In the first year of a child's life, its parents need to devote themselves totally to their newborn.

A woman may have been a busy and active executive juggling a big company, but suddenly she will find that the same amount of effort given to her work is required to attend to one tiny baby. That first year is of great importance for the final development of that baby; a loving maternal presence is essential. By "loving," we mean physical contact in all the various forms of maternal-infant bonding: nursing or feeding, fondling and other manner of showing affection. All the ramifications of future interpersonal relationships will be founded in your baby's first year of life.

NOTES FOR CHAPTER TWO

1. Joan Walker and Morton Walker, *Help Your Mate Lose Weight* (New York: Jove Books, 1978).

2. Tom Brewer and Gail Brewer, *What Every Pregnant Woman Should Know: The Truth About Diet and Drugs in Pregnancy* (New York: Random House, 1977).

3. Joseph William Hazell, "Parental Decisions and Neonatal Health," in *The Bradley Method,* ed. Marjie and Jay Hathaway (Sherman Oaks, Calif.: American Academy of Husband-Coached Childbirth, 1975).

4. Omar Garrison, *Tantra: The Yoga of Sex* (New York: Julian Press, 1964).

5. Morton Walker, *Your Guide to Foot Health* (New York: Arco Publishing Co., 1972).

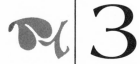

3

Procedures, Problems, and Discomforts During Pregnancy

*If nature had arranged that husbands and wives
should have children alternatively, there would
never be more than three in a family.*
—LAURENCE HOUSMAN

What Happens During Prenatal Visits to the Doctor

It is likely that by the time you become aware your menstrual period has failed to arrive, you are pregnant about two weeks. The need for prenatal care will have begun. Be prepared for a few physical discomforts during the next 267 days. However, the treatment and advice you receive during your prenatal visits to the doctor should offer some relief.

On prenatal visits to your obstetrician's office, the following procedures will probably be performed:

- You will be weighed.
- Your urine will be tested for albumin and sugar.
- Your blood pressure will be measured.
- Growth of the uterus will be measured.
- The baby's heartbeat will be listened to.

These are routine actions. Also on occasion your hemoglobin is checked to make sure you are not anemic. Blood will be taken from your arm for other laboratory tests, including one for syphilis, blood type, German measles immunity, a screening for antibodies and other blood factors, the Rh, hemoglobin, and more.

If you are diabetic, a blood sugar determination will be done regularly; otherwise, this test does not have to be repeated. With a history of kidney disease, urine cultures will be made.

If you have Rh negative blood and are married to an Rh positive husband, there is a possibility your baby may be Rh positive. The fetus will be sensitized to this Rh factor. Then antibodies against the Rh factor will be measured periodically. If you are Rh negative and bear an Rh positive child, you may develop antibodies against the Rh factor after delivery, since the baby's blood can get into your circulation and be a foreign protein. Should you become pregnant again, your antibodies will destroy the second baby's blood, causing the fetus to be progressively anemic.

Significance of Weight Gain and Loss

A mother's weight during pregnancy is very important. The normal pregnant woman should see a weight gain of between twenty and thirty pounds. Weight gain comes on from various changes in your body, such as the addition of the fetus, which adds seven or eight pounds on the average; the placenta forms and is about one pound; the amniotic fluid develops, weighing approximately two pounds; the uterine muscle grows to an increase of about one and a half pounds; an extra blood volume of two pints weighs another two pounds; there is increased weight of the breasts, a minimum of one pound each. These are the minimal weight measurements corresponding to a woman who is five feet tall and normally weighs 100 pounds. A mother-to-be who is six feet tall and normally weighs 160 pounds will put on even more weight. The increases will be mostly in extra dispositions of her body fat.

If a pregnant woman does not gain weight, this is just as bad if not worse than one who gains too much. Lack of weight gain indicates she is neglecting to take in an adequate caloric amount to nourish her fetus and to feed her own body. The common practice of keeping the same weight during pregnancy, which many women once practiced, was doing a great disservice to the baby and to the mother. There is no logical reason to feel proud of beginning pregnancy at 120 pounds and ending at 120 pounds. A new mother who does that has broken down her body fat, caused ketosis in her body, created an abnormal state of body metabolism, and probably has produced a poor mental development for the newborn.

Urine Is Checked for Toxemia and Diabetes

Albumin is a protein substance which is excreted in the urine in cases of toxemia of pregnancy. Toxemia is characterized by swelling of the body, high blood pressure, and toxic substances in the blood and urine. This is a dangerous state primarily for the new mother but may affect the fetus as well. The albumin content of the urine is tested, since its appearance can be a presage of toxemia.

The urine is checked for sugar because the pregnant state is a diabetogenic stress. Altered metabolism during pregnancy puts an excessive demand on the insulin-producing cells in the pancreas. These cells are called the *islets of Langerhans*. If you should have an inadequate ability to manufacture insulin, you could develop diabetes during pregnancy even though you never showed any such tendency before. The diabetes may continue or go away after the pregnancy is over. This manifestation is called *latent diabetes*, a condition brought on by pregnancy and dissipated following pregnancy.

The significance of latent diabetes is that you may at some later time in life, perhaps at age sixty, develop full-blown diabetes. Furthermore, detection of this condition is exceedingly important for the baby's welfare. Diabetes causes you to have a generally continuous higher level of glucose in your serum. The fetus will be exposed to too high a glucose content, which will cause excessive growth. The baby will be overnourished. In order to cope with this overabundant glucose load, the fetus's insulin-producing cells, the islets of Langerhans, will make more insulin to handle the glucose. When the baby is born and suddenly put into a state of normal glucose through formula feeding or breast feeding, its islets of Langerhans will still be geared to produce excess insulin. The baby may then develop a low blood sugar condition as an overreaction to this excess insulin production. Not knowing this beforehand, the hospital nursery staff may not be prepared to deal with resultant convulsions that occur from low blood sugar.

The Need for Blood Pressure Measurements

As we mentioned, one of the symptoms of toxemia in pregnancy is a sustained elevation of the blood pressure. Toxemia should be prevented, if possible, for it harms mothers as well as infants. Unfortunately, it is not entirely preventable, but the effects of toxemia are treatable. Consequently, the earlier your physician picks up signs of toxemia's development, the better. Blood pressure measurements help him to do that.

Should a woman develop toxemia in pregnancy, she must be delivered within twenty-four to forty-eight hours. The baby hopefully will be formed sufficiently to ensure its survival.

Visits for Getting to Know Your Obstetrician

The obstetrician will measure the growth of your fetus at each prenatal visit. He or she may do this with a tape measure or with his or her hands, and will record the expansion of your uterus in centimeters relative to the last visit. This will determine the total volume of your uterus in comparison with other women the doctor takes care of who are in your stage of pregnancy. Such a measurement will reveal if the fetus is growing at an adequate rate—not too little or too much—and will also show if there are twins inside.

All of these measurements and tests are necessary, but possibly the most important reason for you to visit the obstetrician is for the two of you to get to know each other. You are placing yourself in the physician's hands. You will be having a close emotional involvement together. The better you know each other, the better you can interreact when the great moment arrives.

While attending a prenatal lecture in a hospital auditorium, we observed a young pregnant woman in the audience whom we knew. The lecturer was the partner of her personal obstetrician. This young woman came not only to hear the lecture but to observe the doctor who might ultimately deliver her baby. That was a good practice on her part.

In most obstetrical partnerships the patient sees all the associated physicians at separate times. Examination by one doctor on one visit and another on the next will allow for the same amount of encounter with all of them. Prenatal visits usually are planned that way. Appointments will be scheduled to ensure that the doctors know the patient and she knows them. The continuity between visits is maintained by written notes on the patient's chart put there by each examining physician.

The doctor will get to know the patient very well. Why? Well, the doctor asks personal questions of the woman and makes judgments as a professional observer. He makes a comparison of the one patient to about thirty others that he may see that day. The patient only asks questions of the doctor about the pregnancy and the general condition of her and her baby. Intimacy is mostly in one direction—the doctor to the patient but not vice versa.

Our suggestion is to be natural in your relationship with the physician. Be yourself and don't hold back. Don't hesitate to ask any questions and discuss any problems. If you feel afraid, say so! Do not be self-conscious about how you sound. What is most important is staying in good physical and mental condition while having a healthy baby.

Physical Fitness During Pregnancy

The best idea is to be in good physical shape prior to pregnancy, as discussed in the previous chapter. Being in fine physical condition with good cardiovascular conditioning and a strong musculoskeletal system can help you avoid much of the discomfort of the prenatal period. It is perfectly true that when the uterus enlarges, puts pressure on your back, stresses the abdominal muscles, squeezes your bladder, and does other things, you can have some discomfort. You may experience a mild backache and feel the urge to urinate more frequently, since there is less bladder storage capacity during pregnancy. Also some hormones will slow down the intestinal tract so that food does not move along as well, and constipation can occur. However, if you are eating the proper diet with enough roughage, you will not become constipated. The natural fibers will aid in bowel function. Shortness of breath should be no trouble because your good circulation and lung function will take care of this if they are well conditioned. Getting adequate exercise will prevent sleepless nights, too. Your body will relax.

Thus, as we discussed in the last chapter, in a properly conditioned, physically fit woman, pregnancy produces very little discomfort of major significance. The expanding uterus and hormonal changes may be no bother at all. We are told frequently by women that they feel just marvelous during pregnancy—better than they've felt in their lives. These are the ones who are in good physical condition.

Dietary Supplements to Offset Nutritional Problems

The number of miscarriages in the United States each year is estimated to be 400,000.[1] The number of severely mentally retarded children born annually is in the vicinity of 126,000.[2] Estimates have been offered that one child in eight is mentally retarded.[3] In fact, we now face the impact from the more than two thousand known genetic or hereditary diseases. About one person in ten in Western society, or twenty-two million Americans, is seriously affected by a genetic disease, mental retardation, or a birth defect. Approximately 50 percent of the children in hospital beds in this country are lying there because of various types of birth defects, many of which are hidden from view.[4]

Evidence points to such reproductive failure as being caused by the exceedingly poor nutritional environment to which women subject themselves. The effect shows up in the developing embryo, fetus, or newborn, while the symptoms of others may not strike until the fifth or sixth decade. One might wonder why the numbers are not even more staggering. We sound a warning here that the customary American diet is inadequate to support the development of a baby forming in its mother, and dietary supplementation is needed.

Roger J. Williams, Ph.D., discoverer of the B complex vitamin *pantothenic acid*, writes in his book, *Nutrition Against Disease*:

> We know from experimental studies that animals can subsist and reproduce even when their nutrition would be rated *poor*. Poor nutrition can be improved successively to *fair, good,* or *excellent* in many ways: by adding more protein, by improving the mineral balance, and by introducing a better assortment of vitamins in ample amounts.[5]

Babies do not have a chance to develop fully unless the embryonic cells are supplied an adequate amount of every element needed for propagation. Your physician will most likely prescribe prenatal vitamins and minerals. The following are the minimum daily dosages of extra dietary supplements you should be taking while you are pregnant:

Vitamin A—5000 to 8000 IU
Vitamin E—30 to 60 IU
Vitamin C—60 to 120 mg
Folic Acid—0.4 to 0.8 mg
Thiamine—1.50 to 3.00 mg
Riboflavin—1.70 to 3.40 mg
Niacin—20.0 to 40.0 mg
Pyridoxin—2.0 to 4.0 mg
Vitamin B_{12}—6.0 to 12.0 mcg
Calcium—0.125 to 2.0 g
Iodine—150 to 300 mcg
Iron—18 to 60 mg
Magnesium—100 to 800 mg

Also take small quantities of biotin, pantothenic acid, phosphorus, copper, and zinc. The quality of phosphorus should not exceed the quantity of calcium. These are the recommended daily allowances of the United States Government. Though they are inadequate, they are better than no dietary supplementation at all.

What if You Are Pregnant and in Poor Physical Condition?

If your diet does not supply adequate nutrition and you are in poor physical condition, you are likely to experience some of the typical discomforts of pregnancy.

A common discomfort is *dizziness* from insufficient cardiovascular functioning. The direct cause of dizziness during pregnancy is the extra demand of blood required by the uterus. Blood will flow away from the rest of your body. Circulation to the head will decrease if your heart is not strong and your lungs are not supplying enough oxygen for the brain. Dizziness or faintness will come on as a result. To get rid of the dizzy symptom you must exercise. Get in good physical shape.

Headaches arise from a similar phenomenon. The blood vessels of the head dilate and stretch nerves that surround them. This produces pain. Also, many women experience tension headaches from the worry of being pregnant. They feel anxiety that childbirth will be a painful experience. Being in a state of unsureness about what is going to happen, the tension is tied to long-term anxiety.

The best means of reducing tension and ridding yourself of headaches due to anxiety is to become well educated in the childbirth process.

We do not recommend the use of aspirin for relief of headaches. If aspirin or another analgesic must be employed, use it only sparingly. The demonstrated effect of aspirin is that it interferes with blood clotting in the baby, but this is not a clinical manifestation, since a baby does not bleed. The poor blood clotting is a laboratory measurement. It can be avoided by your not taking large doses of aspirin just prior to delivery.

In addition, aspirin may interfere with or slow down the labor process by a poorly understood mechanism.

Indiscriminate Use of Drugs Can Hurt Your Baby

A pregnant woman uses an average of 4.5 different drugs—80 percent not prescribed by a doctor—and unknowingly causes many of the 250,000 annual birth defects in the United States, says Charles Scott, Ph.D., assistant professor of genetics at the University of Utah biomedical test laboratories. The most common of these drugs—laxatives, antihistamines, cough medicines, and antibiotics—are often taken for simple ailments and can cause permanent harm to the child.

"A young girl using tetracycline for her skin since high school gets married and becomes pregnant," Dr. Scott said. "She wants to look nice for her husband so she continues to take the drug, not realizing that it will cause discolored teeth and retarded bone growth in her newborn."

There are four hundred pills on the market which, if taken in excess or with other drugs, cause chromosome damage. The severity of the damage—ranging from mutations causing a change in eye color to an extra chromosome causing Down's syndrome—depends on the dose of the drug and at what point in the pregnancy it is taken. *Down's syndrome* is a condition that includes a variety of infant abnormalities such as mental retardation, retarded growth, flat hypoplastic face, prominent skin folds, protruding lower lip, broad hands and feet, etc. Down's syndrome is also called "mongolism."

"If taken after two weeks of pregnancy, one thing will happen, and if the drug is taken at six weeks, some completely different consequence may result," said Dr. Scott. "In most cases the most severe effect is produced by drugs taken during the first trimester."

Alcohol, a threat to normal chromosomes, can have some remarkable effects on the baby. Dr. Scott recalled how one infant was delivered "drunk from a mother who had a few just before going into labor."

He warned women to be more careful about experimenting with hard drugs. "Men produce new sperm every seventy-two hours, but women are stuck with the same eggs all their lives. For men any damage to the sperm is temporary, but once a woman's eggs are damaged, they stay damaged," the scientist said. Thus, while we don't know of actual instances, Dr. Scott believes that taking hard drugs can cause permanent injury to a woman's ovarian eggs.

Dr. Scott advised couples planning to have a family to definitely abstain from all drugs from several months before to a few months after the birth of their child. He said, "Couples should realize the result of drug taking can be malfunction of the fetus. Mothers, especially, should never take any drugs without specific instructions from their doctors."[6]

Fatigue and Insomnia

In early pregnancy *fatigue* is a universal symptom. Your body is doing a great deal of work to grow the embryo. No matter what your physical state, whether completely fit or an utter wreck, seldom will you feel the same energy and vitality you had before. Normal activities will wear you out sooner when you are pregnant. More rest will be needed, and you should not fight the body's demand for it. Go to bed at 7:00 P.M. if you feel the need. Take a nap after lunch. Just as the growing child needs more sleep, the adult female whose body is expanding from pregnancy does also. Much energy gets expended in the process of growing so that you need to take more rest.

Insomnia may inconvenience you near the end of the prenatal period when you feel uncomfortable from carrying all of that extra weight. You probably won't be able to find a comfortable sleeping position very easily. Before you were pregnant you may have slept in just about any position and rolled over in your sleep without being awakened by the movement, but abdominal enlargement during pregnancy may change all that. Moving from the left side to the right side while sleeping can be a major maneuver. This is a purely physiological and mechanical occurrence and has no particular solution.

Gastrointestinal Distress: Causes and Treatment

Indigestion in pregnancy has two origins: regurgitation of stomach acid and postural pressures. For example, indigestion or heartburn may arise from the gastrointestinal tract moving food along more slowly than usual. Material stays in the stomach longer. The muscles of the gastrointestinal tract are relaxed so that regurgitation of stomach acid into the lower esophagus takes place. Heartburn results.

Later in the pregnancy, pressure from the enlarged uterus compresses the stomach. This pressure prevents full stomach expansion and slows down its ability to empty and push out its digested material. Some of it leaks into the esophagus again, causing symptoms of indigestion.

It will be rare for you to escape these various symptoms of gastrointestinal distress. They are most likely to come on when you are lying down. A horizontal position will cause stomach contents to flow into the esophagus.

To relieve such a condition most easily, we advise you to sleep on two pillows so that a slight tilt is formed. In other words, raise the angle of your head in bed for its postural benefit. You could also raise the bed by putting wooden blocks under the legs of the head portion.

If this mechanical method of relief is insufficient, you can try swallowing an antacid. We specify aluminum hydroxide mixed with magnesium hydroxide antacids as the preferred kind. Aluminum and magnesium hydroxides are safe to take while pregnant and are not absorbed through the intestinal tract. They are gentle, have a prolonged effect, and are excreted totally. Maalox and Mylanta are two brand-name antacids that fit this description. In contrast, sodium bicarbonate antacids such as Alka-Seltzer are *not* recommended. Sodium bicarbonate immediately neutralizes acid and then is absorbed. There tends to be a rebound acidity. The stomach just makes more acid.

Constipation also occurs from a slowing down of the gastrointestinal tract because of the action of hormones during pregnancy. You can best relieve constipation by increasing the fiber content of your diet. Specifically, eat raw, unprocessed bran, a tablespoonful taken with cereal or mixed with orange juice or tomato juice. Eat prunes and figs and the fibers of other raw fruits and vegetables such as celery. Fiber is the antidote to constipation.

Do Not Be Alarmed by Black Stools

Iron is one dietary supplement which requires special attention. Both you and your growing fetus need extra iron, especially in the latter half of pregnancy. The baby stores this iron for his or her needs during the first few months of life.

Your physician may check the adequacy of iron by measuring hemoglobin in your red blood cells. Hemoglobin, an iron-containing protein, carries oxygen throughout the body. Low levels of hemoglobin indicate poor iron nutrition, and the person with a low hemoglobin concentration is said to have anemia. Because the amount of iron needed daily in pregnancy becomes difficult to obtain in the diet, your doctor will probably prescribe an iron supplement just as he prescribes other dietary supplements.

The only problem with iron supplementation, however, is that the iron itself will constipate some women. Furthermore, it will turn stools black. Seeing a black stool and not being prepared for the occurrence could be frightening. Don't be worried! The curious happenstance of black stools from iron ingestion is quite normal.

The truth is that processed foods seldom provide sufficient iron or copper, and supplementation is needed for most pregnant women.

One way to avoid black stools and constipation from iron intake is to eat natural, whole foods that are good sources of the mineral instead of taking an iron or copper supplement. Liver and other organ meats are excellent sources. Dry beans provide protein as well as iron and copper. Use different greens often in place of other vegetables. You pick up vitamin A along with minerals in greens. Choose whole-grain, enriched bread and cereal and the varieties fortified with iron.

Try dried fruits as snacks. Snacks with important nutrients, not just calories, will help to feed your fetus properly now.

Pregnancy is a time to watch your diet carefully. Proper eating helps you to meet your mineral needs after delivery as well as before. Lean meats, fish, and dry beans provide the correct intake of minerals along with protein.

Nausea in Early Pregnancy

Nausea is a common symptom of early pregnancy that has no specific traceable origin. It is probably initiated by sluggishness of the gastrointestinal tract. Added onto this sluggishness is a hunger engendered by your body to provide the embryo with nutrition it requires. You may, as a result, have the contradictory feelings of nausea and hunger at the same time, an odd combination.

Certain foods are said by pregnant women to bring on nausea. Protein, particularly the smell of meat, is a source of complaint. Liquid of any kind also seems to enhance the nauseating sensation. Carbohydrate foods such as raw or cooked vegetables are more tolerable in early pregnancy than are protein foods. Consequently, we recommend that women try to keep some carbohydrates in their stomachs at all times during the prenatal period. Therefore, first thing in the morning you should eat an orange, some carrots, celery, dry whole wheat crackers, or unprocessed cereals such as shredded wheat or Grape-Nuts. Around 4:00 P.M. prevent nausea from coming on by eating carbohydrates again.

If this technique of constant snacking on a carbohydrate food is not sufficient to relieve the nausea, another measure may be employed. A product sold over the counter called Benedectin works effectively. Made by Merrell-National Laboratories, Benedectin's usual dose is two tablets at bedtime unless nausea is severe. Then one additional tablet is taken in the morning and another in midafternoon.

Bladder Pressure and Shortness of Breath

Pressure on the bladder which causes a frequent urge to urinate is a nuisance that comes on a little later in the pregnancy. In Figure 2 you can see that the baby's head is pressing downward on the bladder sac, which is the oval-shaped organ in the abdominal cavity just below the much expanded uterus. Ordinarily, the bladder has room for a little expansion of its own to contain more urine. In pregnancy, it's allowed no room to stretch and thus has to be emptied more often.

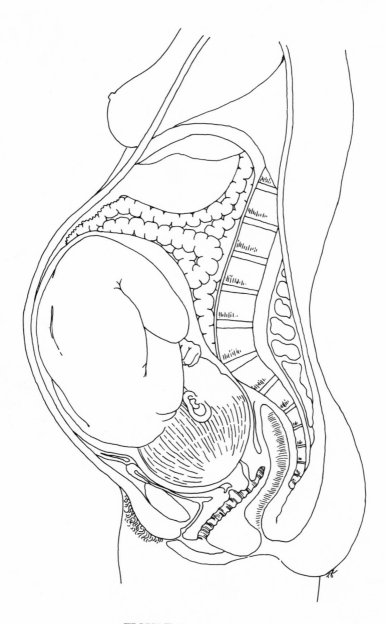

FIGURE 2

The only thing to do is accommodate the urge and pass urine as you feel the compulsion. If you are taking an extended automobile trip, merely stop every hour or so and use available facilities to empty your bladder as needed.

The reason for *shortness of breath* in pregnancy is that blood volume is steadily increased in your body. By the end of the seventh month the total volume of blood has enlarged by two pints. The fluid content of the blood increases first and the more solid particles, such as red blood cells, catch up to fill up this fluid later. While the red blood cells are multiplying, you are likely to have a relative anemia of no great extent. But this deficiency in red blood cells for the quantity of fluid present is reducing the oxygen-carrying capacity of the blood. This will give you the feeling of shortness of breath. Also, an increased blood volume will make your heart work harder, and the need to breathe more vigorously will come from more stringent heart action.

Not only that, but the growing uterus puts pressure on the diaphragm just under your lungs. In Figure 2, you can see that all of the internal organs are displaced by the growth of the baby and uterus. The digestive organs including the intestines are pushed upward. In turn, they press against the diaphragm, which separates the lungs from the digestive cavity. The space for the lungs is lessened. They cannot expand sufficiently, so that one feels a shortness of breath and the need to breath more frequently. If your physical condition is good, this shortage of breathing capacity will not be a bother to your baby to any extent. You should be able to adapt to it. Being out of condition, of course, will cause you more discomfort. That is another reason that preparation for pregnancy is so important. Get in good condition physically as soon as possible, as we have advised in Chapter 2.

Leg Cramps and a Stitch in the Side

Painful cramps or aches may occur in the legs as a result of a buildup of lactic acid in the leg muscles. When muscles are working they require more energy for metabolism. Their metabolic rate of energy expenditure is increased, and this metabolism takes place in the presence of oxygen. However, when the blood flow to the muscles is insufficient for the amount of work they are doing, the muscles tend to try to get along without oxygen. Then lactic acid accumulates and the muscle starving for oxygen cries out in pain. You will feel *leg cramps*. This is the very same problem that is experienced by long-distance runners as they near exhaustion.

During pregnancy your muscles are working harder than usual to carry a greater load. In addition, you have the problem of a swollen uterus pressing on pelvic veins. The blood flow through these veins slows down and your leg muscles may suffer from oxygen starvation. Lactic acid buildup and the need for oxygen produce more leg cramps.

Just as with shortness of breath, the prevention of leg cramps comes from being in the best physical condition possible. Get your muscles in good shape in advance of pregnancy. If not prepared, the only treatment to offset the leg cramps is rest or stretching out the affected leg and massaging it with a good rubefacient liniment available at the drugstore.

A *stitch in the side* is nothing more than oxygen starvation in a muscle in that area. The round ligaments supporting the increasing weight of your uterus become overworked. Similar to leg cramps, the treatment for a side stitch is rest or massage. Mild heat may help, too.

How to Accommodate Backaches

All *backaches* for anyone, pregnant or not, result from a certain instability of the spinal column and weakness of its ligaments. Because of this ligamentous weakness, the back muscles are forced to hold everything in place. If they are overstretched, these muscles go into spasm and produce full-blown back pain. Muscles in good tone, however, will not spasm and will stay strong to help stabilize the weakened spinal structure.

Pregnancy puts extra stress on the back structures since you are steadily growing in a forward direction to throw your body off balance. The back muscles must pull on the abdominal wall to hold the torso upright. This pulling will make you become somewhat swayback. To complicate matters, the hormones of pregnancy cause the ligaments of the pelvis and lower back to soften. Softened ligaments tend to make the whole skeletal structure less stable and the muscles are called upon to work and strain. Therefore, they protest through pain.

Your most effective action to avoid backache again should begin before pregnancy with suitable exercises and body conditioning. But being pregnant now, and still developing backaches despite previous preparations, the best thing to do is employ as good posture as you can. Do not allow yourself to become swaybacked. Sit in firm chairs that give strong back support. If you have to stand for a long time, such as in washing dishes at the sink, raise one foot on a short stool.

Lifting the leg as little as three inches will relieve pressure on the back muscles and prevent swayback. And you should sleep on a firm mattress that offers good support. If your mattress is soft, put a plywood board under it for firmness.

NOTES FOR CHAPTER THREE

1. N. J. Eastman and L. M. Hellman (eds.), *Williams Obstetrics* (New York: Appleton-Century-Crofts, 1961).

2. J. B. Richamond, "Mental Retardation," *Journal of the American Medical Association.* 191:243 (1965).

3. A. Levinson and J. A. Bigler, *Mental Retardation in Infants and Children* (Chicago: The Year Book Medical Publishers, 1960), p. 29.

4. J. L. Wilson, *Congenital Malformations* (New York: International Medical Congress), 1964.

5. Roger J. Williams, *Nutrition Against Disease* (New York: Pitman Publishing Corporation, 1971).

6. "Even Aspirin Taken by Mother Can Hurt Baby, Doctor Says," *Los Angeles Times,* July 28, 1974.

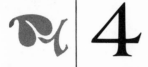

4

Labor: The Long and the Short of It

To me, labor was totally different. . . . I thought it was extraordinary—concentrating on it and observing it as an outsider. . . . It was just what happens when something expands and changes . . . [evolves and explodes]. Ah, something strange, definitely, but not pain.
—CATERINE MILINAIRE, Birth

How to Almost Calculate the Birth Date

Some women have their babies easily and naturally without putting much effort into childbirth preparation. They are rare. The majority of women require advance instruction that includes techniques of breathing control and relaxation to maintain the greatest comfort.

Following forty weeks of pregnancy the baby is ready to come out into the world. You calculate the approximate date by adding nine calendar months and one week to the first date of the last menstrual period. While most newborns arrive within a week before or after this date, they cannot be relied on to do so. It is not unusual for an infant to let you know he or she is ready to be born at a time somewhat different from your calculation. In fact, only about 5 percent of all births occur on the calculated due date; 35 percent take place five days before or after; and the remaining 60 percent happen even earlier or later.

Each Pregnancy and Delivery Is Unique

During her labor, one of our patients pleaded vehemently not to have the usual enema administered. When asked why, her tearful reply was, "I'm afraid you'll drown my baby!"

A young Chinese woman was told by her grandmother the sex of her unborn infant. The wizened old lady had grasped her granddaughter's wrists and checked the pulses. Then she read from an ancient text that said: "When the pulse of the left hand is rapid, without fading, the woman will give birth to a male child." Somehow she was correct. The woman gave birth to a boy.

There is much misinformation connected with giving birth. You do yourself a great disservice when you enter childbirth ignorant of your own anatomy and physiology. By being well informed and educated about what the birth process involves, you will know better how to handle yourself and remain in control during labor. You can be assisting the actions of the greatest of all midwives—Mother Nature!

Giving birth is one of those rare and important moments that makes life worth living. The joy, anticipation, and excitement are exhilarating. No other emotions can compare. The excitement can be destroyed, however, if fear and ignorance play too big a part. The result could be loss of control. Knowing what to expect next helps you to retain control and avoid much discomfort.

Do you wonder how you will know you are in labor? Maybe you have inquired when to call the doctor. One of the most common questions asked of obstetricians is, "Will I recognize when I'm ready?" Since each pregnancy and delivery is unique, even women who have given birth previously may be misled by the signs.

Labor is an unpredictable thing. For example, one of our patients, an athletic woman who had been the local tennis champion, should have delivered swiftly. She was in very fine health, but her labor was long and fruitless and required medical assistance. Yet a second patient, pampered and flabby, had her baby in very little time and with a minimal amount of effort. No one can tell you exactly what will happen. Labor can be easy or difficult. It may be short or it may be long.

Labor That Was Short

Mrs. Channing Brown had labor that took a relatively short amount of time—perhaps too short. "I got to sign my own son's birth certificate, since I was the one who delivered him. It was really quite a

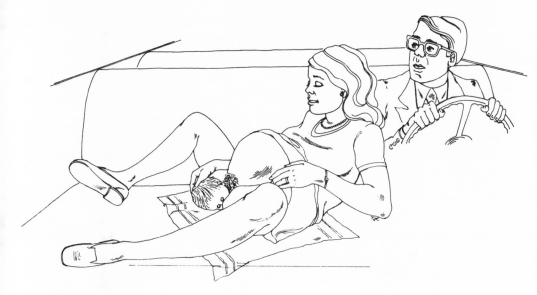

FIGURE 3

surprise," Mrs. Brown said, her big dark eyes twinkling while she related her experience in delivering her own baby while en route to the hospital. "I really thought I could make it, but it just happened too fast." Baby Stafford Brown arrived somewhere near Exit Six on the Connecticut Turnpike at 3:10 A.M. The Browns live in Monroe, Connecticut, usually a forty-five-minute drive from the hospital.

"It's one of those things every expecting mother worries about, and I'm no exception," she said. "We moved quickly after my water broke at around two A.M., and the labor pains started right up.

"We made the trip in less than thirty minutes that morning, with my husband racing down the turnpike at speeds of seventy-five to eighty miles, and no one stopped us," Mrs. Brown explained.

"We were only three miles from home when the pains were coming three minutes apart, but when we got past Norwalk, I thought I could make it. We were moving along well and it would have taken more time than we had to stop and look for a police escort. Our only thought was to reach the hospital so the baby could receive proper care," said Mrs. Brown.

She sat on the front seat of the car while Mr. Brown drove. They approached the hospital exit on the turnpike. At that moment she knew there was no way of holding back any longer. "There was no fear, and I wasn't that uncomfortable. I realized I could handle it and decided to let nature take its course. When I said, 'Here it comes,' my husband thought I meant another labor pain, but the baby's head was coming out," she said.

Her husband looked over and was shocked. Then in an assuring voice he kept repeating, "You're terrific! Oh, how beautiful you are."

Mrs. Brown said, "The next moment the baby emerged totally. I guess I was extremely lucky, for he started breathing and crying almost immediately so that I knew everything was all right."

Instructions about emergency techniques for birth incidents that she remembered reading in a first aid book had said that the less one handles a newborn the better; just keep it warm and close to the mother. "I had the forethought to bring along a towel, and I just held him in my lap," she said. "It was strange. I had this child for the first fifteen minutes or so and didn't know if it was a boy or girl. It was dark and I couldn't tell. I didn't think that we should stop under a streetlight to find out. I just held him close to me unknowing, till we reached the hospital."

Young Stafford Brown weighed seven pounds and was perfectly healthy.

Such extremely short periods of labor occur perhaps once in every two hundred births. Hospital emergency staffs habitually list at least one baby born a year en route to their hospital, generally in the ambulance or in a police car.

Labor That Was Long

Mrs. Patricia Orsino's labor was very long. Her husband, Paul, said it was an uphill battle all the way. She went more than eighteen hours with contractions just five or ten minutes apart the entire time. For two weeks in advance her small valise had been packed for the hospital stay; she was that anxious to experience her first childbirth in the natural way—awake and aware. Paul and Patricia were prepared by prior attendance at childbirth education classes. But her long labor arose out of an anatomical difficulty—the birth canal was too narrow. "Our baby was born with an exceedingly pointed head," Mr. Orsino said. "The head was compressed by the birth canal walls and took a few days to assume its normal shape.

"We had gone out to a party that evening—dancing and all," explained Paul Orsino. "We arrived home about midnight and were just dozing off when everything started. It was a surprising experience—not something I had expected."

Mrs. Orsino agreed that the way her labor began was startling. She described the scene: "At two A.M. on Thursday, May 13, 1971, I was awakened by the breaking of my bag of waters. My husband immediately telephoned the doctor who instructed us to go to the hospital. As we drove the fifteen-minute distance, contractions began five minutes apart. I mistakenly believed I might have an easy time, but as I was prepared and examined in the labor room, I learned that I was still only dilated the same one and a half fingers I had been for two weeks. I was in labor when the doctor arrived at eight o'clock that morning.

"He checked my stagnated progress and said the bag of waters from above, rather than below, had broken first, and it was 'dry labor' that I was experiencing. I hadn't known that a water bag was located at the neck of the cervix, too."

It was a severely intense labor—contraction after contraction—no letting up at all. The new mother became exhausted, but she refused analgesics and wanted to go all the way without outside help.

"They got me out of bed to pace the labor room and squat during each contraction. This was something I hadn't learned to do before, but it's very handy to know; the baby is pushed down into the birth canal with the contraction working for you," Patricia Orsino said.

"Still in labor at five P.M., the doctor and my husband discussed cesarean delivery but decided to give me one more hour . . . and another one, too. Around six thirty P.M. I felt the first urges to push—and push I did—straight through until eight fifteen P.M. Into the delivery room we went and three good pushes later, it was a boy, Paul Thomas Orsino, Jr., born eight forty-four P.M."

How Labor Is Handled in Foreign Cultures

For every woman labor and delivery are a time when one's body becomes a stranger. That stranger takes over the childbirth function. Any loss of control is, at some level, frightening. You may meet that fear by ignoring it; by learning about breathing, massage, and exercise; by stoically saying, "This is the way childbirth is so I'll just accept it."; or you may elect to have some form of anesthesia. Being unique, labor will put demands on you that might not have been anticipated. One must rise to the occasion.

For instance, an experienced mother in our practice, about to deliver, called for her baby to appear. She rooted, "Come on out, boy! Come on out to play baseball with daddy!" The newborn arrived swiftly, and to everyone's surprise, she gave birth to a boy.

Another frightened woman in labor who knew nothing about what to expect lay on the delivery table crying woefully, "Oh, Lord! Jesus Christ have mercy on me!" Each woman confronts labor in her own way.

Women in labor in foreign cultures also go through long and short periods of arduous activity to give birth. Enlightened doctors in the Solomon Islands of the South Pacific believe they have the ideal method for coaxing out reluctant newborns. It is said that when a woman is late giving birth, natives take the father down to the low tide mark and tie him to a stake. At the same time, the mother-to-be is taken to an overhanging bluff to watch the tide come in.

The idea is that she will force herself into final labor before her husband drowns at high tide. According to reports from the South Pacific, they haven't lost a father yet.

Among some Mexicans and Spanish-speaking women of the U.S. Southwest, a rope arrangement is worn under the breasts that is knotted over the umbilicus to ensure a safe delivery.

Food taboos to ward off evil during delivery are common. In Polynesia, eating an egg with a double yolk is thought to practically ensure the birth of twins. Polynesian women avoid eating joined fruits along with double yolks because they don't want to have a twin pregnancy.

Some cultures associate the eating of strawberries with the strawberry birthmark that affects a few babies.

Looking at the full moon while pregnant is said in certain Latin-American lands to give rise to crippled or deformed children.

In a few societies pregnant women are housed in a pregnancy hut, separate from men. Perhaps this long standing practice has been the cause in this country to exclude husbands from the delivery room. Birth customs of the past do occasionally determine current procedures during labor.

What Labor Is and Is Not

Labor may be defined as the onset of regular uterine contractions which increase in frequency, duration, and intensity leading to the forced expulsion of a fetus from the uterus at the normal termination of pregnancy. Labor has been divided into three stages. The *first stage* is the period of dilation of the cervical opening of the uterus (mouth of the womb). The *second stage* is the actual expulsive effort, beginning with the complete dilation of the cervix and ending with the delivery of the infant. The *third stage* begins with the delivery of the infant and ends with the complete expulsion of the placenta (afterbirth).

Although the methods of childbirth have changed in many ways, the labor process has not altered since Eve brought forth Cain and Abel. But one thing certain is that labor cannot be forecasted as to time, place, risks, and severity. Thomas P. Kerenyi, M.D., director of the perinatology division of Mount Sinai Hospital in New York, said, "There is no foolproof method for prediction."

Dr. Kerenyi believes even a normal woman with no signs of risk or complications should give birth in a hospital instead of in a homelike maternity clinic or at home attended by a lay midwife. He said, "The biggest problem is how to identify the high-risk population. . . . Some high-risk women, such as diabetics, you know about ahead of time, but you can find young women in the ideal reproductive age group, perfectly healthy, thinking very positively about pregnancy and child-birth, who develop problems that there was no way to anticipate, not only during labor but in the delivery room right in the middle of birth."[1]

The Three Signs of Labor and Delivery

The baby lies waiting in your uterus, which is a large, pear-shaped bag filling the abdomen almost to the level of the ribs. The placenta is attached to the inside wall of the uterus. Connected to the placenta are the thin but tough membranes, making an enclosed uterine lining, and containing the watery amniotic fluid which keeps the baby warm, protects it from bumps and pressure, and allows it to move about.

There are three signs of labor and imminent delivery. These signs include the "show" (a pinkish vaginal discharge), the powerful contractions themselves, and the rupture of membranes (breaking of the bag of waters). One or more of these three signs indicate that it is time to notify whomever it is who will be in charge of the delivery of your baby.

In labor, the cervix, which is tightly closed during pregnancy, must become thin and open. The lower part of the uterus, the cervix, and the upper part of the vagina must be drawn up by the uterus past the infant's head. At the same time the head must move down through the pelvis and the vagina. Then the baby and the placenta and membranes will be free to be delivered from the uterus. From this first stage of labor onward, the vagina is called "the birth canal."

To understand why and how the three signs of labor and delivery take place, you should know a little of the anatomy of the uterus. Its upper part is made up of strong active muscles; the lower, less active part is continuous with the cervix. The cervix is the thick, fleshy opening that leads into the upper part of the birth canal. In turn, this leads to the birth outlet. At the lower edge of the birth outlet is the perineum, which is the skin and muscles between the birth outlet and the anus.

The Bloody "Show" of Mucus

A thick discharge tinged with blood, the "show," indicates that the mucous plug, which closes the mouth of the uterus during pregnancy has been painlessly dislodged as the cervix begins to dilate. During pregnancy the mucous plug, like a stopper on a bottle, keeps germs from entering the uterus and affecting the fetus or the mother. The bleeding comes from uterine pressure on the tiny blood vessels of the cervical membrane. The amount of show varies from individual to individual. Less commonly there is a gush of bloodstained mucus. Sometimes there is a persistent leakage of clear fluid from the vagina, which indicates that the membranes have broken.

The cervix will have begun to thin out. Some frequent but extremely mild contractions probably are happening now. Pressure forces out bloody mucus from a large number of glands lodged in the walls of the cervix. When the labor is well advanced and the dilation of the cervix opening is seven to ten centimeters, there can be quite a heavy blood show. This is a useful sign and indicates that the first stage of labor is coming to an end.

In explaining the feeling of full dilation to ten centimeters (about four inches), one of our patients described it as the same sensation you would get by putting two fingers on each side of your mouth and pulling, pulling, pulling until you can't pull any longer. Then give one more big pull until your lips are hooked back behind your ears. That is how it feels to be fully dilated.

Breaking of the Bag of Waters

Muriel Lomax, a woman near the end of pregnancy, was singing Christmas carols onstage in a choir before a large audience. She and her forty fellow choir singers were wearing long black robes. Suddenly Muriel felt a stream of liquid running down her left leg, and she realized the bag of waters within her uterus had broken. For a few moments she was panic-stricken. She forgot the words of the song she was singing. Then Muriel took hold of herself and vowed to remain calm. It was obvious that she should do something to catch the waters puddling at her feet, but walking away from the recital would have been too distracting for the audience and the other singers. She kept her cool and just stood there voicing the words. When it was over, Muriel dribbled off the stage and telephoned her doctor for advice.

Breaking of the bag of waters is nothing more than a lot of liquid running out of your vagina. It may be embarrassing if it happens in a public place, but the trickling is not dangerous. If you are at home, get a big Turkish towel, put it between your legs, and just sit quietly for a few minutes until the initial gush is over. Then let your doctor or nurse-midwife know what has happened.

Amniotic fluid is released with the painless breaking of the bag of waters. As described, it may gush suddenly or trickle steadily from the vagina. Membrane rupture is a normal beginning of labor, but only about 10 percent of all women experience it as the first sign. In about 50 percent it occurs during the last hours of labor. Sometimes the bag of waters remains intact, and the person delivering the baby may rupture it, quite painlessly, to speed the labor along.

The water bag can be broken rather easily with the use of a sterile orange stick. The stick's sharp point penetrates the bag, which resembles a balloon filled with water. When the puncturing is done, liquid leaks out and you feel the joyous release of pressure. The bag's breaking by itself usually indicates that labor is going to begin sometime within the next forty-eight hours. In fact, about 90 percent of women will go into labor spontaneously within twenty-four hours of its rupture.

What is the bag of waters? It is nothing more than two membranes which surround the fetus. Some women have membranes stronger than others. The membranes have a few functions. They prevent infection from getting into the uterus, keep the umbilical cord from falling down, but more importantly, they offer a buffer to the baby's head. As it grows and gets ready to come out, the fetus is surrounded by a cushion of waters continuously. Even as it moves through the birth canal, the membranes and water serve as a good dilating wedge for the cervix and vagina, making them open wider!

It is the opinion of top experts in childbirth that the membranes are best left intact until the very end of labor. Individuals anticipating giving birth at home should be aware that rupturing the membranes to expedite the labor is not recommended. One of the dangers is that artificial rupturing may cause compression of the umbilical cord by the sudden gushing of waters and loss of their shock absorption quality.

An associated condition that should be warned against, especially for home delivery, is bright red bleeding heavier than a menstrual flow. Blood running down a pregnant woman's legs is an abnormal situation and could indicate one of two dangers: *placenta praevia*—a placenta that has implanted itself low over the mouth of the uterus; or a *placenta abruption*—a placenta which has begun to separate from the uterus too early. Expert obstetrical treatment is required for these two conditions.

Contractions of the Uterus

Most women beginning labor will feel some mild, somewhat irregular contractions of the uterus. The contractions may not be particularly noticeable but rather are similar to insignificant menstrual cramps. This occurs from the uterine muscle being affected by changes in the various functional systems of your body: the endocrine, nervous, humoral, and psychological systems. Uterine contractions are *involuntary*. Their action is independent of your will.

Contractions of the uterus feel like abdominal cramps which start slowly and radiate from the lower part of the back to the front of the abdomen. The gradual tightening of uterine muscles rises in intensity, reaches a peak, then relaxes slowly—similar to the rising, cresting, and falling of waves on the shore. At first, the muscle hardening may last a few seconds and be twenty minutes or more apart; but the contractions gradually become more frequent, regular, and stronger.

Our suggestion is that you not pay much attention to the beginning contractions, since they are likely to go on for an average of fourteen hours, and even longer for first babies. Later, the powerful contractions will have gradually forced the baby down into the cervix and cause that passage to stretch to a diameter of about four inches to allow the baby to pass into the lower birth canal. Therefore, try to relax completely during the early labor contractions. If you are relaxed, cervical dilation is enhanced. Breathing slowly and deeply will allow you to feel more comfort during these contractions.

False labor frequently resembles true labor, but instead of progressing to harder and more recurrent contractions, the false labor decreases in intensity after a few hours, and it will disappear. It occurs at irregular time intervals and may be relieved simply by changing the position of your body. False labor occurs during the late months as a result of the fibers of the swelling uterine wall gently contracting and relaxing at irregular intervals to exercise the uterus and improve circulation.

With the first baby, when your contractions occur every five minutes, and have continued every five minutes for one hour, you will know that you are in early labor. A contraction makes your abdomen feel as if it is a tightened drum. The tightening and hardening of muscle tissues may arise from the back and come to the front. Some women say it feels like a stomachache. The contractile wave may last for forty to sixty seconds and become progressively stronger.

Dilation of the Cervix

The length of time that it takes for the cervix to dilate from being completely closed to four centimeters open is an individual condition. Also it may be influenced by medications such as narcotics, sleeping pills, and alcohol.

Figures 4–7 illustrate the degrees of cervical dilation ranging from zero centimeters to six centimeters.

Figure 4 shows no dilation of the cervix. It is closed and labor has not begun.

Figure 5 depicts cervical dilation at two centimeters. The opening is occurring passively under the power of the uterine muscle which is above it. This is called *effacement* of the cervix, a thinning out and flattening of the neck of the uterus. Effacement is at its maximum when the cervix is thinnest. In the ideal situation effacement takes place prior to a woman's going into labor.

Figure 6 indicates the cervical opening at four centimeters.

Figure 7 shows the opening at six centimeters. Here, contraction of the uterus at its upper portion is pulling on the connective tissue fibers at its lower end. They are lifted up. The vagina stretches out and gets larger like a plastic tube. Once a woman has passed four centimeters of dilation, she is said to have entered the active phase of cervical dilation. From this point the cervix thins and expands at one and a half centimeters an hour, on the average.

Near the end of pregnancy one can walk around for two or three weeks dilated two or three centimeters without having any further elements of labor; actually no labor pains! Only your gynecologist will know from the internal examination given. You can be dilated with symptoms or without. It varies from person to person.

Sometimes dilation measurements are given in terms of the number of fingers of dilation rather than in centimeters. This measurement terminology is poor practice, since each examiner's fingers vary in size. The finger of a male obstetrician could be as large as two centimeters in diameter. An inch equals 2.54 centimeters.

The only thing that can stop cervical dilation once it has entered the active phase is the oversize of the baby's head relative to an undersize of the mother's pelvis. This is a complication that usually requires cesarean section.

The "Transition"

The term *transition* is frequently used in obstetrics to indicate the moments just preceding birth when the woman is told she can push out the baby. It is an artificial term designating an artificial period that

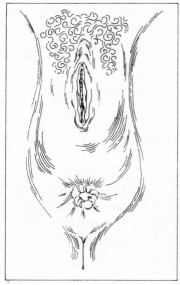

FIGURE 4

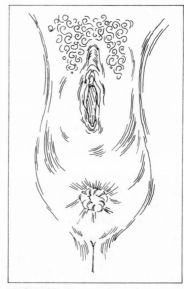

FIGURE 5

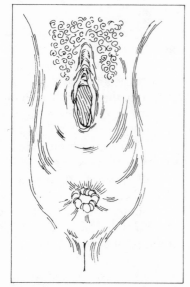

FIGURE 6

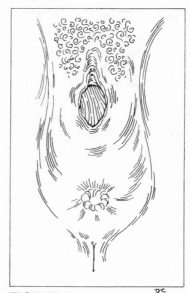

FIGURE 7

was invented as a convenience by that pioneering obstetrician of Great Britain, Grantly Dick-Read. It is a term not generally recognized or used by the obstetrical branch of medicine in the United States. We consider the moments of transition irrelevant, since the woman in labor will falsely anticipate them as the time she can let go. Yet the person delivering her baby may still wish her to remain in control and follow directions—to push or hold back from pushing. We suggest the term not be used even though it is well ingrained with some childbirth educators.

The end of the first stage and the so-called transition may be a difficult period emotionally. There is often no precise point at which it is possible to say that the first stage is over and transition has begun. The interval between labor and delivery (the second stage) is gradual. The cervix may be fully open but the baby's head must come farther down into the birth canal and the upper part of the birth canal must be drawn up by the uterus. For this reason, we repeat our recommendation that it would be wise to do away with the term, *transition*.

Expulsion of the Newborn

Once the cervix is fully dilated and can no longer be felt around the baby's head, the second stage of labor has begun. This is the stage of expulsion of the newborn. It is accomplished by the continuing contractions of the uterus which press on the baby and the voluntary efforts of the mother bearing down to push out the baby. The baby begins to descend into the *birth canal*, which we have explained is just another name for the stretching vagina.

As the mother pushes downward, she performs an action akin to the feeling one has with a bowel movement. Much energy is expended. There is resistance from the inherent lack of elasticity of the birth canal. The mother feels a friction caused by the baby's head against her vaginal walls. A woman with strong abdominal muscles will have a shorter second stage of labor than one who is flabby and in poor physical condition. The flabby woman cannot push as hard because of insufficient muscle tone.

Pushing in the second stage of labor is the hardest work a woman might ever have to do. Although she has put out a great deal of energy already, she often finds renewed strength to push her baby out.

In the second stage an end is in sight and the pressure of labor changes. The mother feels better! Unless the second stage goes on for an hour; then she begins to feel discouraged. Her energy gets diluted. She will begin to wonder why her baby has not come out yet. That is the time when her attendants and coach must reinforce her with kindness and encouragement.

The second stage of labor ends with the birth of the baby. When she has pushed out the baby's head, most of her work is then ended. The shoulders follow rapidly and then the rest. Normally the newborn is laid on the mother's abdomen for her to see it, touch it, stroke it. All the while the obstetrician observes the baby to ensure that it is breathing well. It may not cry. It does not need to cry. Nevertheless, when the newborn does cry the anxious mother and father feel a lot better.

The umbilical cord attached to the mother inside and to the newborn at its umbilicus continues to pulsate at the rate of the infant's heartbeat. The person who has delivered the newborn can assess its condition by feeling how readily and strongly the umbilical cord is pulsating. Then pulsation will stop on its own and the cord can be clamped and cut. The pulsing beat ends because the baby's own circulation pattern takes over. Pulsation of the umbilical cord may continue from within a few seconds of birth to as long as five minutes.

The Third and Final Stage of Labor

After birth of the baby, expulsion of the placenta takes place. This is considered the third stage of labor. The placenta is attached to the wall of the uterus. Normally with the contraction of the cervical neck of the uterus after delivery of the baby, the surface area of the uterine wall decreases and shears the placenta from its attachment. The uterus expels the placenta into the upper vagina, where the mother can very easily push it out.

Following this expulsion the uterus continues to contract, closing all of the larger blood vessels which have been supplying the placenta during the pregnancy. That is the end of labor. Some authorities on the birth process call this contraction of the uterus to shut down the placental blood supply the *fourth stage* of labor. Certainly it is the final internal act of the mother in bringing forth her baby.

Over the next six weeks the uterus continues to contract and shrink. Ten days after the delivery the uterus is no longer an abdominal organ. Sufficient contraction and shrinkage take place so that it almost completely returns to its prepregnancy state inside the pelvis. The mother may experience afterbirth pains which are strongest during the first few days following delivery. These pains will be felt the most when she nurses, as a result of the baby's suckling. Breast feeding causes the nipple to react and force the release of a hormone from the pituitary called *oxytocin*. Oxytocin simultaneously accomplishes expression of milk from the breast and contraction of the uterus. Mothers who nurse consequently help their uterus return to normal size more efficiently.

NOTES FOR CHAPTER FOUR

1. Rita Kramer, "Revolution in the Delivery Room," *The New York Times Magazine,* July 11, 1976.

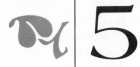

5

Nonparticipating Childbirth

She will come in a radiance of new-made skin,
in a room of dying men and dying flowers,
in the shadow of her large mother,
with her books propped up and her ink-stained fingers,
lying back on pillows white as blank pages,
laughing: "I did it without words!"
—ERICA JONG, *Loveroot*

The Human Species Goes On

She walks alone, stopping as each wave of pain contorts her body. In stopping, she pants for breath. This is a familiar path to the bush. She has given birth to three babies already—this Enga tribeswoman of New Guinea—with no prenatal care, no monthly checkups, and no spotless delivery rooms. There were never any competent doctors and nurses to attend her while she birthed her child in a squatting position over an open trench. If she bleeds much this time, the Enga woman will jump up and scurry about until the bleeding stops. The method has worked before.

She will cut or bite through the umbilical cord, shave the infant's head, and place the afterbirth high in a tree if it is a boy, which will ensure that the boy will grow up unafraid to climb trees. For a girl, the afterbirth will be tossed away or buried. The Enga woman knows to stay in the bush with her newborn for a month so her husband will not be contaminated. If she has twins, the second baby must die. If she has a difficult delivery, she will die.[1]

The human species goes on generation after generation in New Guinea, despite these primitive conditions of childbirth. Women have

managed to reproduce even amid superstition, ignorance, and the unknown. In every society childbirth has been surrounded by customs
and rituals. It is that way in our modern Western society as well. For
example, the practice of removing a healthy baby from his or her
mother's room during their hospital stay has been our birth custom.
Perhaps it should be changed with more expanded use of *rooming-
in*—the baby remaining with its mother continuously for feelings of
attachment to take place.

The Origin of Nonparticipating Childbirth

Nonparticipating childbirth is the current custom for the majority
of births in this country. It probably began November 4, 1847, in
Edinburgh, Scotland, when Sir James Y. Simpson, a physician, discovered the anesthetic value of chloroform. He applied the anesthetic
to relieve the sufferings of childbirth.

For the first person who inhaled chloroform fumes for childbirth, it
took effect immediately. She was made unconscious and delivered
within twenty-five minutes. The cry of the baby did not wake her and
much time went by before the mother woke up at all. She slept, in
fact, for three days. Upon finally opening her eyes she said the sleep
was quite restful and now she could go on with delivering her baby.
During the time the mother had been "put under," all her labor pains
had stopped. In no way was the new mother aware she had already
delivered her child.

A week later Dr. Simpson published his report about this successful
childbirth employing chloroform to do away with the pains of labor.
A violent medical controversy arose over use of this technique. He
was denounced far and wide in circulated printed pamphlets and in
speeches from church pulpits. Later, opposition to chloroform anesthesia for childbirth dissolved when Queen Victoria accepted it for her
own delivery.

Antiseptics began to be used in the 1890s. The furniture pieces in
lying-in wards were washed with a solution of carbolic acid. The
rooms were then left unoccupied with open windows for several days.
Straw bedding was banned because of its uncleanliness and higher
cost. Patients in labor admitted to hospitals were given rectal enemas
of soapsuds, and they received vaginal douches of bichloride of mercury.

The mother was given no choice. It was all part of the nonparticipating childbirth procedure, done automatically—a new technology
introduced into obstetrics.

The bichloride of mercury was an antiseptic. The most frequent infection in those days was caused by hemolytic streptococcus, the same germ that causes strep throat today. Douching is never done now, since modern medical doctors believe that the normal flow of blood and serum (the *lochia*) that comes from the uterus after delivery has its own cleansing property and washes any bacteria away from the uterus. To douche, we now know, merely pushes bacteria into the uterus. The trend is toward more natural methods in the current practice of obstetrics. The earlier technology was contrary to nature and a woman's natural lochia discharge.

As time progressed, antiseptic methods and chloroform anesthesia were used more and more. Technology increased. In one well-known case, a California physician gave chloroform to a woman whose unborn baby was in a transverse position. The mother was frightened and claimed she did not need chloroform because she had given birth to nine other children. Finally, as labor progressed, she agreed to take the anesthetic. When she awoke on the dining room table, she discovered she had delivered not one baby but three. Afterward she vowed she would never take that stuff again![2]

Modern Anesthetic Techniques

The commitment of physicians to relieve pain runs a close second to the saving of life. It is their oath. For that reason, modern anesthetic techniques have been perfected even for such a natural event as childbirth. The basic tenet held by obstetricians and nurse-midwives or other persons assisting the laboring woman is to be the hand that helps. This includes making childbirth as painless as possible.

Although education and preparation for giving birth may reduce your discomfort markedly, pain may remain to a high degree. Perhaps you prefer not to bear it. It is one of your options. Since you are the one giving birth, you have the right to choose the method that is right for you. It is far better to request and accept anesthesia and welcome the comfort it affords than to suffer needless discomfort you feel unable to withstand.

All techniques of childbirth cataloged in this book are dedicated to birthing a healthy baby with as much comfort to mother and child as possible. The transcendent objective of obstetrics, including midwifery, is that every pregnancy culminate in a healthy mother and healthy baby. It further aims to minimize the discomfort of pregnancy, labor, and delivery.

Various improvements have been developed in the twentieth century to allay the discomfort associated with childbearing. Some put you to sleep. Most do not. A few involve analgesic techniques that utilize barbiturates to induce drowsiness. Scopolamine is used only occasionally now to produce amnesia for the childbirth events. A narcotic analgesic such as Demerol or morphine is given. At one time gases such as ether or nitrous oxide were inhaled for the actual delivery.

There are various limitations of these sedative or analgesic or anesthetic techniques. All of the substances used to sedate the mother also pass through the placenta to sedate or anesthetize the baby as well. In order to cope with this problem, physicians experimented with the various drugs in the first half of the twentieth century. They discovered that lower doses of the anesthetic substances had to be used. They found antagonists for the narcotics in the 1940s. Antagonists were administered to the mother just prior to delivery or to the baby just after birth in order to wake them up from a sleepy state.

Improvements of anesthesia techniques came in with the development of the spinal anesthetic. A further refinement came along with the lumbar epidural or caudal anesthesias. We feel compelled to state that none of these methods should be administered routinely. The woman in labor must be allowed her options—make the decision to have an anesthetic assist if the discomfort becomes too great. Or choose not to. It is her body and her baby. Consequently, she should have at least a cursory knowledge of the different forms of analgesia and anesthesia. For that reason, we describe here the various types available along with their characteristics.

Lumbar Epidural Anesthesia

The spinal fluid and spinal column are encased in a sac called the *dura*, and nerves coming out of the spinal column penetrate this sac. When local anesthetic is injected into a potential space that exists between the ligaments of the bony vertebrae and this dural sac, epidural anesthesia takes place to block the sensory nerve fibers. The motor fibers that call for you to move and push out the baby are not affected. This anesthetic technique merely relieves the pain. You are not paralyzed and you will have motor function. Your ability to push and move remains, but there is no pain. It is possibly one of the more enjoyable methods of anesthesia.

So why is it that more publicity is not given to this technique? Epidural anesthesia is difficult to attain because of the great amount of training required to get the anesthetic solution exactly in the right place. Your doctor must be highly skilled with a needle and syringe. Not everyone is.

The advantage of epidural anesthesia is that it can be administered fairly early in labor, as early as when the cervix is four centimeters

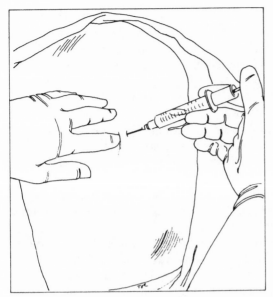

FIGURE 8

FIGURE 9

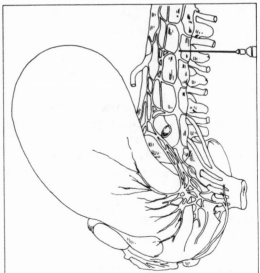

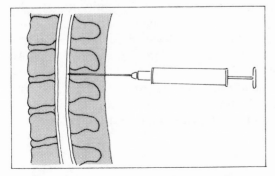

FIGURE 10

dilated. This is the time you are just beginning to get into the active phase of labor and discomfort has started. Epidural anesthesia can be maintained throughout the rest of labor and for the delivery itself. When done properly, you will be completely free of pain, yet awake and able to move about.

Shown in Figure 8 is the first step: some local anesthetic is put into the skin of the back by injection.

Next, a fairly large needle is inserted through the locally anesthetized skin into the spinal column. Through this needle a fine plastic tubing called the catheter is fed through the needle into the potential space present between the vertebral bones and the sac that encloses the spinal column. This step is shown in Figure 9. Also shown are the nerves coming out of the spinal column that penetrate the sac of the column called the *dura*.

Figure 10 shows the anesthetic being forced through the catheter into the potential space between the vertebral bones and the sac that encloses the spinal column. This epidural space is outside the dura. The anesthetic blocks the nerves emerging from the spinal column, and you feel nothing from the lumbar area down.

The technique for epidural anesthesia has a few other disadvantages besides being difficult to perform. For one thing, it may not work correctly. Blockage may affect some nerves and not others. The laboring woman could have pain relief just on one side of her abdomen.

Furthermore, if the needle is improperly positioned, the anesthetic might escape into the spinal fluid itself to create a total spinal anesthesia. This could be quite dangerous. The nerves of the autonomic nervous system thus being blocked, the patient will sustain a profound drop in her blood pressure. This drop would be detrimental not only to her but to the baby. Blood pressure must be monitored by the anesthesiologist every few minutes while the anesthetic is going in. Epinephrine is given for a blood pressure drop. This drug makes blood vessels contract and brings the pressure back to normal.

Such an epidural anesthetic administration requires the attendance of an anesthesiologist every moment the patient is laboring. If she is in labor for eight hours, she must be attended the entire time. Obviously, this professional attention would entail enormous expense. And because she feels no sensation in her uterine area, the woman has no urge to push once the cervix is fully dilated. Forceps will possibly have to be used for the delivery.

Too much relaxation of the muscles around the vagina is a frequent result of epidural anesthesia. The muscles fail to maintain their tone and the natural muscle resistance against the baby's head is lost. It is this muscle resistance which causes the baby to rotate into the proper position to be expelled. When this muscle tone is lost, the baby will frequently hold a transverse position in the uterus with its head sideways, or even maintain a posterior position with the face up. To be delivered the baby must face downward. However, the mother under epidural anesthesia feels none of this and just waits for the obstetrician to do his or her work. The operative manipulation with forceps because of overly relaxed vaginal muscles is no benefit to the baby at all.

Saddle Block Spinal Anesthesia

In saddle block spinal anesthesia a local anesthetic is injected into the spinal cord, and the anesthesia takes effect downward. As we mentioned, this injection rids you of pain and eliminates muscle tone as well. Thus there is less resistance in the birth canal to your baby's head passing through, since your vaginal muscles are relaxed. You are awake and may choose to push as an assist to delivery, although this is not a prepared form of participation. This is another method where you are awake but feel no discomfort.

Illustrated in Figure 11 is the extent of anesthesia supplied by this pain-relieving technique. Pain and motor function are removed from the pelvis and the area of the body that would be in contact with the saddle if you were riding a horse. This is the reason for calling it the *saddle block*.

Figure 12 shows the penetration of the needle into the back at the level where anesthesia is desired. The skin has been numbed with a local anesthetic prior to the penetration of the longer needle.

Figure 13 shows the needle injected directly into the spinal fluid. The anesthetic takes hold of the spinal cord and allows operative delivery with forceps or an episiotomy to be cut and sewn without your feeling it at all.

The saddle block is very good anesthesia for an operative delivery with forceps. It allows for the forceps to be applied with ease, gets rid of pain, permits the baby to be rotated and extracted, if required. An episiotomy can be cut and sewn without your feeling it at all. The technique is easy to administer, takes effect at once, and is relatively safe. The blood pressure does not drop dramatically.

The saddle block spinal anesthesia's big drawback is the headache afterward that affects about 10 percent of women taking it. The headache could be present for four or five days after childbirth simply from leakage of the spinal fluid out of the puncture site where the injection

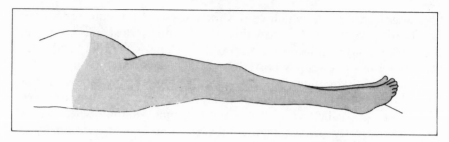

FIGURE 11

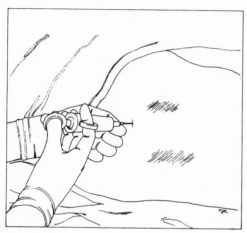

FIGURE 12

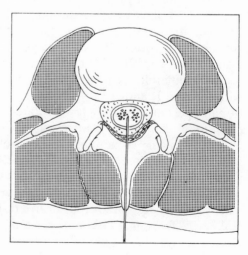

FIGURE 13

was made. Such a leakage lowers the pressure of the spinal fluid at a time when the spinal fluid pressure seems to require an elevation during childbirth and just afterward. The headaches can be extremely uncomfortable. They strike anytime the new mother sits up. She must remain quiet on her back sometimes as long as ten days afterward.

Aside from the headaches, spinal cord anesthesia is useful, safe, and a happy way to give birth. It is administered close to the time of delivery. If it is given earlier than that, labor stops. Perhaps the woman is not fully dilated at the time. Then she will not become dilated fully until the spinal anesthetic wears off. As indicated, there are advantages and disadvantages with use of any of these techniques.

General Anesthesia

General anesthesia involves inhalation of a gas. The entire body and brain go into a relaxed state. The patient falls asleep and feels no pain while muscle function is abolished and uterine contractions slow down. The one big advantage to the use of inhalation anesthesia for childbirth is that it completely gets rid of all sensations and anything can be done to expedite the birth, including episiotomy, forceps delivery, abdominal pressure, and manual extraction of the placenta. Some women prefer this technique, since they have no desire to know anything that is going on. Childbirth becomes the doctor's job entirely.

Disadvantages do exist. Inhalation anesthesia is accompanied by the danger of vomiting while under the anesthetic. This regurgitation is a significant cause of morbidity and mortality of women in labor.

Also, general anesthesia can only be employed right at the end of labor just before the baby is expelled; otherwise, the uterine contractions slow down. The newborn will be affected by the gas along with the mother. The only way to minimize the gas effect on the infant is to give it at termination of the first stage and get the newborn out rapidly once the mother is asleep. The type of gas is a factor, too. Some anesthetics reach the infant sooner than others.

Paracervical Block Anesthesia

The popularity of *paracervical block anesthesia* is fading into history, but it is still used in some areas. The nerve fibers arising from the uterus can be reached through the upper vagina. A local anesthetic injected into the cervix at its lower quadrant will block pain fibers and relieve pain caused by cervical dilation. It is a simple and effective technique and does not slow down labor to any significant degree.

However, paracervical block anesthesia does present problems which have caused it to fall into disfavor. Along with the nerve fibers run all the blood vessels going into the uterus. The anesthetic may be absorbed very rapidly into these blood vessels and invade the placental circulation. By crossing the placenta, the fetus will be affected by the anesthetic which can have a toxic effect.

Measurements have been taken of the amount of toxic anesthetic agent in the fetus approximately twenty to thirty minutes following its administration to the mother's cervical area. Simply going through the vagina and pricking the infant's scalp will indicate an anesthetic blood level that is damaging. The fetal heart rate will slow inordinately as a consequence. Even with delivery soon after administering the anesthetic using the paracervical block technique, the infant will have trouble breathing. The potential hazards of local anesthesia into the cervix outweigh the benefits, and the technique is being abandoned.

The Pudendal Block

While painful contractions of the uterus continue during the second stage of labor, most of the pain of delivery is transmitted through the pudendal nerve. The peripheral branches of the pudendal nerve provide sensory innervation to the perineum, anus, and clitoris. It can be blocked from carrying pain by injecting right next to the nerve fibers that carry pain a local anesthetic of the type used in dentistry. Anesthesia is administered through the vaginal wall down to the pudendal nerve.

This pudendal block is of no value for analgesia during labor but may be employed for vaginal delivery. From the standpoint of safety, local infiltration anesthesia is preeminent. The advantages are:

1. There is practically no anesthetic mortality.
2. Fetal mortality or deprivement of oxygen from the direct effect of the anesthetic agent is absent.
3. Administration is usually easy. It can be administered by the person delivering the baby and does not require an anesthesiologist. Thus, local anesthesia is suitable for home and hospital delivery.
4. Uterine contractions are not impaired.
5. There is no need to hurry through an operation.
6. The toxic effects are minimal.

One problem with the pudendal nerve block is that the blood vessels and nerves travel together, and it is possible to place the anesthetic agent into the pudendal artery. That can cause shock to the patient's system—even death. The trick is to ensure that the needle point is not in the artery by aspirating the syringe (making sure no blood comes back into the syringe before injecting). The artery is frequently hit accidentally, however, and the hole in the arterial wall lets blood leak into the surrounding tissues to create a hematoma, which is a collection of blood around the vagina. Otherwise, this is quite a safe technique. The least amount of local anesthesia is administered into the skin of the lower vagina and the skin between the vagina and anus just prior to delivery.

Twilight Sleep

Twilight sleep is produced by administration of scopolamine. This drug eliminates pain of delivery by putting the woman out and, when used in sufficient dosage, takes away any memory of pain. There is no "measurable" effect on the baby with use of this anesthetic.

A shortcoming of scopolamine is that under full doses the mother will behave in an irrational fashion. The drug annihilates a lot of her normal inhibitory actions. Scopolamine is hardly used anymore even though it takes rapid effect. Within twenty to thirty minutes of taking the injection the patient falls asleep between labor pains. She occasionally moves around restlessly and sometimes cries out with contractions.

Demerol and Tranquilizers

Demerol is often employed in conjunction with 0.4 milligrams of scopolamine. Their combined effect is similar to that produced by the taking of barbiturates and scopolamine. They take away pain exceedingly well.

Demerol may also be used alone. Its disadvantage is the effect apparent in the baby. A full analgesic dose of Demerol sufficient actually to get rid of the mother's pain entirely will have a depressing effect on the infant's respiratory center. Is there danger? Yes, some. The baby will have difficulty in breathing upon first entering the world. Demerol will cause your baby to appear sleepy for the next two or three hours.

On the other hand, tranquilizers create a reduction in the baby's reactions that last as long as four or five days. From reduced reactions, a baby won't suckle as well—will be less responsive altogether. This may result in a lower scoring index for the Apgar tests, which we will discuss in detail in Chapter 24.

Doctors place great value on Demerol and therefore have made some adjustments in its use. The patient becomes the beneficiary when she needs its narcotic effect. A full pain-relieving dose of Demerol is 200 milligrams. This is the dose used for a person with a kidney stone, one of the most painful conditions anyone can have. Such a high dose of Demerol will relieve the pain of the passage of the kidney stone, but given to a woman in labor could adversely affect the newborn. To get around this problem in obstetrics, Demerol doses are reduced to 75 milligrams or less. This is a full analgesic dose and still does not influence the baby's breathing to any extent.

Vistaril, hydroxyzine hydrochloride, is a tranquilizer that potentiates the effect of narcotics such as Demerol. It allows a woman in active labor having a fair amount of pain to relax while objectively allowing the cervix to dilate more readily. Vistaril tends to ease the whole of labor if administered when the cervix is dilated four or five centimeters.

Psychological Motivation for Having Anesthesia

When you visit your obstetrician who determines you are pregnant, a question that invariably will be asked, almost mandatory nowadays, is: Are you interested in taking prepared childbirth classes? Your affirmative reply does not obligate you to have *no* anesthesia if you desire it. Perhaps you will be surprised to learn that it was solely in response to the public's demand for relief of pain in labor and delivery that physicians such as Sir James Y. Simpson developed the many techniques that exist. But as we have stated earlier, times and practices have changed. Medical technology for childbirth may be lessening.

We believe that the relief of pain itself, although desirable, does not justify the use of anesthesia methods which themselves may be dangerous. The proper psychological state for the mother throughout the antepartum period and labor is a more valuable sedative. If you are free of fear and feel complete confidence in the person who is to deliver your baby, you will enjoy a relatively comfortable first stage and second stage. You will require a minimum of medication or none at all. Your psychological preparation for giving birth is that important.

The pains of childbirth have been the stock and store of intimate conversations among women since time immemorial. Many young women approach the birth of their babies in dread of the ordeal and that is the reason for the rise of nonparticipating childbirth. It is no easy task to dispel this age-old fear. The psychological motivation for having anesthesia is strong. The emotional aspects of labor are as real and significant as their physical counterparts. And absolutely unquestionable is that your attitude toward your delivery has a major influence on the ease of your labor.

Nonparticipating Childbirth Is Contradictory to Natural Childbirth

To eliminate the harmful influence of fear in labor, a school of thought has developed emphasizing the advantages of "natural childbirth." This is contradictory to the technology of nonparticipating methods. Natural childbirth requires participation, usually with preparation. We will discuss several techniques of preparation for birthing in some chapters that follow.

Prepared childbirth entails antepartum education designed to eliminate fear and make the process as comfortable as possible, through exercises in relaxation, muscle control, and breathing, and adroit management by the mother throughout labor with skilled reassurance by the person giving assistance.

Grantly Dick-Read, who began the movement away from technology and back to methods of natural childbirth, was a proponent of labor and delivery without anesthetic aids if possible. He called his techniques "painless childbirth." However, with natural childbirth, most women still experience some discomfort, and analgesics and anesthetics are not withheld when they are indicated.

The psychological motivation for anesthesia will be lessened if the patient enters labor with a high morale, a positive attitude, and the knowledge that her helpers are fully skilled and giving total attention to her needs and desires. We concur with Oliver Wendell Holmes who said:

> The woman about to become a mother, or with her newborn infant upon her bosom, should be the object of trembling care and sympathy wherever she bears her tender burden or stretches her aching limbs. . . . God forbid that any member of the profession to which she trusts her life, doubly precious at that eventful period, should hazard it negligently, unadvisedly, or selfishly!

NOTES FOR CHAPTER FIVE

1. Shirley J. Nicholson, "Birth Customs Reveal Society's Values," *Health* 18: 16–20 (July–August 1973).
2. Nicholson, "Birth Customs."

6

Prepared Childbirth— the Father Gets Involved

Larry and Bonnie Experience Childbirth Together

Larry Underwood left his wife for a few minutes to smoke a cigarette. He had been timing Bonnie's contractions faithfully for several hours. In the father's waiting room we had a chance to talk.

"I wanted to go into the delivery room during all four of her pregnancies," he said, "but with our first child the hospital didn't allow it. A husband-as-helper was a new concept to that section of the country at the time. I assisted Bonnie with the others though."

"What draws you to participate with your wife in the childbirth experience?"

"I want to know what's going on instead of sitting out here for three or four hours wondering if she's all right. I have to know how everything is coming out. I think I can help my wife. She wants it that way, too."

"How can you help her?"

"By just being there and offering reassurance. Letting Bonnie know that she is doing a good job is a great help. Then, for her to see me takes away anxiety about whether I'm smoking too much, pacing the floor, and in a sweat with worry. It's—it's moral support, if nothing else."

"Do you give her physical support as well?"

Larry shrugged, "Not too much. I don't have that much to do. Just time the contractions—tell her if she is breathing correctly—massage her back if she needs it to relieve the ache. You see, I'm as much a part of creating this baby as Bonnie is. I kind of want to give birth along with her. It's no obligation, no duty. This is something I'll feel good about just doing it. I never had fear that I'd get sick at the sights and sounds of childbirth. Rather, I've felt excitement and joy every time. Seeing my child born is really something! I can't keep a smile off my face during the whole procedure. Even with knowing the whole time that my child is growing inside Bonnie, the significance of it comes home to me when I see it actually delivered before my eyes. I know very well—that's my baby!"

Bonnie and Larry Underwood had a healthy baby boy whom they named Christopher.

General Advice for New Fathers

Studies have shown that participation by the father in his mate's labor and delivery fosters a special attachment similar to that between mother and newborn. Daddy will feel a special tie between himself and the baby whom he has witnessed being born.

General advice given to new fathers suggests that as part of your education you should attend parent-preparation classes with the mother. Such classes are great confidence-builders. They get you actively involved in the pregnancy and birth, and help prepare you for oncoming fatherhood. You'll learn how to coach and support your mate during labor and delivery so that childbirth is a truly shared experience. It firmly binds the couple relationship.

There are many complexities involved in becoming a father. No doubt you will react differently from the next fellow, but here is a piece of advice every father can use: have confidence in your own importance. Fathers profoundly affect their children's lives from the very beginning. Your involvement will make a vital difference in the kind of person that baby becomes.

The Father's Function Before Baby Is Born

Inasmuch as paternal behavior is a learned behavior, you might think of yourself as engaging in a new educational experience. You will have deep emotional feelings, of course, and many anxieties arise in advance of fatherhood. In truth, the anxieties will be there whether you are a first-time parent or a well-practiced veteran. Typical questions you could be asking are: "How can I assist in the additional household chores? Will I be able to bathe the baby—or feed it—or diaper it—or pay for it?"

Beginning anxieties will be relieved more easily by your attendance at prepared childbirth classes, hospital demonstrations of baby bathing and feeding, and by a prenatal visit to the pediatrician. Yes, visits with the pediatrician of your choice prior to the infant's birth will be most reassuring. Questions about infants usually get answered during such visits, and prenatal interviews with pediatricians are becoming more common.

We have observed a frequently confronted conflict by some fathers. They lack feelings of confidence in themselves to manage their prenatal role. Fatherhood is not altogether instinctive. Training is necessary. Taking steps to get educated about parenting and becoming a helpmate to the mother, perhaps before conception even takes place, is the way to build self-confidence.

You can help a great deal by encouraging your mate to make prenatal visits to the doctors involved. Show your interest. Accompany your spouse during those visits; question the physicians; listen to the baby's heartbeat; make sure the mother-to-be does everything she is told to do for her benefit and the baby's. Maybe maintain your own proper nutritional program along with her. Exercise together. And generally keep in good physical condition. Do all the many things good for you and her in body, mind, and marriage.

Talk openly so that any underlying worries will surface and can be solved between you. Discussion will be good for your relationship during this time of family transition.

Sometimes stresses exist before the birth of a new baby that require balancing the needs of the mother, father, and siblings. Interpersonal relationships within the family are bound to change. It will be the father's responsibility to work toward strengthening the family unit by taking charge and preparing the other children to receive their new brother or sister.

By anticipating your mate's needs, you can develop a supporting role and make her life easier. Being tired, harassed, or preoccupied with work or sporting events will really interfere with the attention you should be giving her. Therefore, you should cope with your wife's mood changes, altered sexual desires, and other emotional variations by sublimating your needs to hers. Our suggestion is to court her again as you did before you were married. Take her out for visits with friends and relatives or for other forms of entertainment. Her mood changes usually arise out of her boredom with routine.

There will be little variation in your sexual relationship in the first trimester of pregnancy. Then her sexual interest diminishes somewhat during the second trimester and is much diminished in the last trimester. By wooing your wife as a lover, your sex life may be prolonged. Besides this, being more loving will help to keep up her morale and make the pregnancy easier, at least mentally.

A Husband's Actions in the Labor Room

A husband is the finest tranquilizer and the most effective pain reliever for his wife in labor. The several jobs he must perform in the labor room, while seemingly trivial compared to the event about to take place, are exceedingly important to a woman at this time. Some of the actions taken by the husband-coach are:

1. Furnishing sips of water to freshen her mouth
2. Giving back rubs to relieve the discomfort of muscle tension
3. Providing counterpressure against back labor
4. Acting as her spokesperson to the health professionals in attendance
5. Filling out necessary hospital forms
6. Supplying ice chips for her to suck on
7. Adjusting the bed and bedclothes
8. Changing into hospital greens during the first stage of labor so as not to be separated from her during the second stage
9. Offering verbal encouragement to her
10. Timing the contractions and the intervals between them
11. Remembering and employing all the techniques for prepared childbirth both of you have learned

As the attentive mate, you may make the judgment that the pain of labor is too great for your wife to stand. Or you may recognize that the joy and thrill of working hard together is the main goal so that you will help her stave off the need for analgesia. Your observations will be valuable. And your techniques to ease the burden of labor will help your mate to relax.

Peter Swain Higle, a natural childbirth educator in the Bradley Method of Husband-Coached Childbirth, says: "The teamwork atmosphere set up between you for relaxation is the most important. One of the techniques a man can use is imagery relaxation. With use of this imagery technique you conjure up the picture of a favorite place where both of you have been that was extremely tranquil. By describing that place, you can evoke a peaceful feeling. This might help to reduce your wife's discomfort during a contraction.

"Being well-practiced as the coach makes labor for your mate much easier," added Peter Higle. "You have to be well rehearsed, and this rehearsal puts you on the same wavelength with your wife. It is a finely tuned conditioning that both of you have—one to the other.

"The main requirement to be an effectively coaching husband, however, is an honest desire and commitment to help. It isn't the kind of thing that can be laid on *all* prospective fathers. Going only halfway into any one of the prepared childbirth courses won't do at all. If you have love and caring, though, you will possess the equipment to go all the way and help your spouse and newborn achieve a happy, unmedicated birth."

Father's Role as Mother's Helper

We have suggested that the father's function as mother's helper actually starts before labor ensues. In the months preceding birth your helping begins with making sure your mate keeps up with her exercises, continues to eat following the best nutritional principles, and does not run for an aspirin at the first feeling of headache or backache. In short, your role as husband-coach starts early in the pregnancy with words and actions of loving reinforcement. For instance, you must hold her back from eating pizza, hot dogs, white bread, and candy with the use of reinforcing words of advice and not by eating those junk foods yourself. Do the physical conditioning exercises along with your wife. They are just as beneficial for men as for women. Coaching involves mutual participation from the start.

Your most significant physical contribution, however, will be to help relax her through the most difficult times of labor, the really severe contractions. If you have ever watched a dog or a cat in labor, you will note how the animal goes into complete passivity between the contractions. It conserves every bit of energy possible and uses it for confronting the next contraction. You can help your mate accomplish the same thing by using the verbal imagery described by Mr. Higle. Talk her into a semisleep state. No matter what is going on around you—nurses coming and going or doctor visiting to check—continue to express yourself with soft words of relaxation, encouragement, and love. Read her the following poem, "Relaxation," by Rhondda Evans Hartman, for it is ideal as a means of creating imagery:

Let your whole being
Sink slowly, slowly, slowly.
Feel your muscles
Becoming limp and loose and comfortable
Drifting or floating
Relaxed and comfortable.

Warmth and heaviness
Is spreading through your body.
The baby in your uterus
Is warm and heavy.
Feel warmth and heaviness
Spreading from the baby to your abdomen, hips
Thighs, knees, lower legs, ankles
Feet and toes.
Slowly, the lower half of you
Is loose and limp
Warm and heavy.

The upper half of you awaits its turn.
Slowly release, let go
Warm and heavy
Limp and loose
Let every cell absorb and enjoy
Spreading up back and front
Chest and shoulders.
Arms and hands and fingers, let go.

As your neck releases tension
Your head slowly shifts and becomes
More and more relaxed.
Nearer and nearer that comfortable state of
Relaxation.

Erase the worries from your brow
Eyes loose but closed
Eyes and all around eyes
Limp and loose.

Cheeks loosen and droop
Jaw drops
Tongue is loose in your mouth
Lips part slightly.
Warm, heavy and comfortable.

Deep, slow, heavy breathing
Breathe in and out slowly
Abdomen up and down slowly.

Limp and loose
Warm and heavy
Comfortably relaxed.

In your mind's eye

Hold a softly purring kitten in your lap
    while sunshine warms you both.

Listen to the laughter of children
    sledding on a crisp sparkly snowy hill.

Ride a bicycle on a lazy autumn afternoon
    Hair blowing in the wind.

Sit before a roaring snapping fire
    with a red shiny apple ready to eat.

Watch a robin build her nest
    Weaving string and straw with precision.

Lie on the warm sand near your love
    Watching the waves roll in.

Limp and loose
Warm and heavy
Comfortably relaxed.

Another function for you as labor coach is to apply manual pressure to the mother's body when needed. At least a third or more of laboring women will feel contractions in the back. If this is the case for your mate, the coaching job will include providing firm counterpressure to the small of her back. The need for this pressure could go on for hours. The fetal position in the uterus sometimes puts pain on the mother's spine, so counterpressure from the outside provides a welcome relief.

Giving such back-pain relief can be exhausting for the man, especially if he has not prepared for the event. We recommend that you practice in advance by performing isometric exercises by pressing against a wall in your home.

As the laboring woman's coach, your job also entails being her consumer spokesperson. She will be less able to demand her rights and voice her needs while preoccupied with contractions. For example, if the attendant should try to give the mother-to-be an internal examination during a contraction, it will be in your province to request that the examination wait until the contraction is done. If she does not want her pubic area shaved but the hospital practice usually includes one, you can refuse the shave on behalf of your mate. In other words, the husband-coach is his wife's communicator. He verbalizes to the nurses the agreed-upon instructions made in advance with the doctor. Nobody wants surprises; surprises bring on anxieties which will increase the discomforts of childbirth. We will have more to say about labor-coaching for husbands in Chapter 10.

Does Male Chauvinism Get in the Way of Helping?

Being mother's helper in her time of travail is not for every man, as indicated by Peter Higle earlier in this chapter. Some men continue to hold the attitude that giving birth is strictly woman's work. They apparently classify this bringing forth of a newborn in the same category with washing dishes, scrubbing floors, and darning socks. A few men feel this way as a result of their upbringing—male chauvinism that comes from prior conditioning.

Enrollment in a course of prepared childbirth tends to change this chauvinistic attitude. You are shown that childbirth is something more vital than personal preferences. Men learn of paternal-infant bonding and overall fathering, in addition to preparation for helping mother at labor and delivery. In classes, fathers-to-be spend time exploring how it is going to feel being a parent. They talk among themselves and relate to their new responsibilities. Our observation has been that a man who prepares for fatherhood and participates in prenatal activities becomes a better parent. Just as there is a mother-child attachment that takes place within the first hour of birth, there is father-child bonding simultaneously. And these feelings begin in the prenatal period. We will discuss this parent-infant bonding further in Chapter 21.

Male chauvinism could get in the way, perhaps at first. But an eye on the final reward of feeling a closer tie to the baby will overcome any uncaring kind of thinking. The roles of masculinity and femininity are merging in our society. Changing an infant's diaper or feeding, bathing, and comforting him or her are no longer being considered woman's work. They are all part of parenting.

Does Prepared Childbirth Turn a Woman into a Militant Feminist?

The couple who prepares for natural childbirth should experience a closer emotional bonding between themselves. It is not a sexual thing. Rather, it just means that the woman trusts her man so much she would want him for her labor coach. In turn, the man accepts that trust and assures his mate that he will provide his unfailing support. In childbirth, undoubtedly, he will have to deal with the least attractive part of his mate as she goes through the effort of labor.

Predictably, what intimidates some men at the outset of going into prepared childbirth classes is militant feminism. Their worry is that the techniques of unmedicated childbearing will in a way turn their wives more toward the women's liberation movement. Many husbands want no fires lit under their wives that will cause them to feel superior. They could not tolerate such an attitude. Consequently, a few men will feel suspicious of prepared childbirth classes and wonder if their women will be turned into those kinds of militant feminists.

The various childbirth preparation techniques do raise a woman's realization of her own worth. Through having such a drugless experience, awake and aware, she comes to know that she is emotionally and physically tough. Such a realization may tend to threaten a lot of men.

We suggest that attendance at childbirth preparation procedures should not scare you. Go ahead and find out if your male ego will be endangered. We know that it won't. Open your mind and grow as a couple from the experience. It is a worthwhile sharing—a labor of love.

Advice from a Participating Father

Dennis F. GiaQuinto, a husband-coach who helped his wife in labor and delivery, offers words of wisdom about the childbirth process. He says: "My advice for other fathers-to-be is *preparation*; be aware of the series of events and their possible deviations. Try to think ahead as to the ways your wife may react to birth events. Only in this way will you be the best help.

"During labor, time can seem endless," said Mr. GiaQuinto, "and your encouragement, understanding, and direction may mean the difference between success and failure when using the natural child-birth method—especially in a really long labor.

"Of itself, being in the delivery room means that birth is near. There you will merely be repeating in a concentrated form what you've already learned and what the doctor says should be done. You will hope that your wife reacts mechanically, following the sound of your voice. In my own case, our very rapid labor and delivery made my usefulness limited, but I was ready if the labor had been longer. The longer your wife has to work, the more useful you'll be as a coaching husband," he concluded.

The Reality of Paying for Childbirth

In her text, *The Complete Book of Absolutely Perfect Baby and Child Care*, author Elinor Goulding Smith jokingly says: "It sometimes happens, even in the best of families, that a baby is born. This is not necessarily cause for alarm. The important thing is to keep your wits about you and borrow some money."

Alas, the reality of paying for childbirth does arrive eventually. It is best to be prepared and put money aside for the event.

A normal pregnancy and delivery costs between $1000 and $2000, of which only a few hundred dollars is paid by medical insurance. Childbirth is an "elective procedure" as designated by many insurance policies. The prices for obstetrical care vary around the country, but the cost of professional services generally runs high.

For example, in the metropolitan New York area hospital costs run more than $1300 and an obstetrician's fee is around $700. That high cost is one major reason young couples are turning to midwives—delivery and prenatal care costs only $500 on the average. Childbearing centers such as the Maternity Center Association in New York City charge $750 for the entire childbirth, including prenatal care, labor, delivery, and postnatal care. There is no separate hospital cost. A home birth costs much less; and many lay midwives are paid in groceries, or charge nothing.

Our recommendation is to rebudget for household expenses to enable you to pay off all or a large part of the doctor and hospital bills during pregnancy. It is easier to face the big moment that way. Try to cut down on regular living expenses before you take on extra work. Working two jobs may be a financial solution, but we believe that your emotional involvement with your wife and the time you spend with her are especially important now. Try to avoid getting wrapped up in money worries; instead spend your time in preparation for being mother's helper.

Health Insurance for the Infant

At its forty-sixth annual meeting held in mid-November 1977, the American Academy of Pediatrics discussed the high costs connected with care of newborns who are endangered by a health problem. Crushing medical bills for babies are not uncommon today. Sophisticated medical technology is able to sustain life in imperiled infants who in the past would have died. Parents can be relieved of much of that economic burden by health insurance policies which cover their child from the moment of birth.

But even with recent passage of a law to cover the newborn including the first thirty days of life, you cannot assume the costs will be paid. Policies written and purchased prior to the newborn insurance legislation do not have to be altered to conform. Consequently, as part of your financial protection for childbirth and any complications sustained by the baby, discuss early coverage with the person in charge of insurance benefits at your place of employment. If there is insufficient time to effect a change in a group policy, George M. Wheatley, M.D., past president of the American Academy of Pediatrics, urges taking out personal coverage for that period. The extension of aid for the newborn will probably add between sixty cents and one dollar to your insurance premium.

Coverage from the moment of birth is totally in keeping with the basic principles of insurance, Dr. Wheatley said. "If a child is born prematurely and possibly with a congenital defect, the situation is both unpredictable and catastrophic."

The academy makes the following suggestions about health insurance for the infant:

- Review your policy carefully. If it seems to be inadequate, discuss it with your agent or with the individual in your company or union responsible for insurance. Inform colleagues of inadequacies. Insurance benefits are important components of labor negotiations.
- If you are not covered, purchase health insurance immediately. Coverage for dependents is available to single parents as well as couples. (According to Dr. Wheatley, a personal family policy may cost between $1200 and $1400 a year.)
- If your policy does not include ambulatory sick care, agitate for

it with your representative. If you hold a group policy which may take time to change, purchase insurance on your own to cover important gaps.

- If you expect a baby and your policy has an exclusionary provision, take out additional insurance for the uncovered period of time.
- Notify your carrier within thirty days of the baby's birth, providing the infant's name, birth date, sex, and your insurance policy number.

Health insurance protection for the newborn becomes part of the reality of paying for childbirth. Acquiring such protection becomes part of the many roles a father plays as mother's helper.

In a healthy marriage the husband should help wherever he can. Janice Wehmann said, "Oh, I'll tell you what got me through seventeen hours of labor—having Warren there. If he hadn't been there to coach me and time my contractions, I don't think I could have given birth naturally. Why, do you know once he got so tired while counting seconds he went twenty-eight, twenty-nine, thirty, fifteen, sixteen . . .? Yes, he counted up to thirty and dropped back to fifteen! I thought, oh, it's almost over, and I looked, and the poor guy was timing with his eyes closed."

Warren Wehmann admitted, "Yes, I was practically asleep. This was like six in the morning after Jan had labored for twelve hours. To stay awake, when she didn't need me for coaching, I stitched her needlepoint."

"He didn't make any mistakes either," said Janice.

7

The Dick-Read Approach to Natural Childbirth

*Natural childbirth! Me? In the early months of
my pregnancy when my doctor suggested the
possibility of such a delivery I nearly fainted
with terror. I'm the sort of person who defensively
informs the dentist of my "low pain tolerance"
while asking for Novocain. As the weeks passed
I gave little thought to natural childbirth.
Then in my fifth month of pregnancy, my
doctor casually said, "Gretta, you should be
starting the exercise class soon."*
—GRETTA P. ESTEY, *American Journal of
Nursing*

Natural Childbirth Fulfills a Primeval Emotional Need

Grantly Dick-Read, M.D., has demonstrated that childbirth can be
a joyful and satisfying experience. Before he died, Dr. Dick-Read
perfected and taught others to accomplish "the beautifying of the maternal conscience . . . not only for the mother herself, but for her
home, the community and the nation."

The Dick-Read approach to natural childbirth is based on *inter-
rupting the fear-tension-pain cycle*. The mother's fear leads to tension
which then causes pain. The pain then leads to more fear. You will be
able to reduce fear, perhaps eliminate it altogether, by providing your-

self with information about the childbirth process. Education about what is happening offers a deconditioning away from earlier fears, myths, and misconceptions.

With use of any kind of childbirth method, the physical safety of mother and infant is a primary concern. In natural childbirth, the primeval emotional need of a woman to feel satisfied and fulfilled in her unique ability to bring forth life is also achieved. By employment of the Grantly Dick-Read approach, childbirth without fear is accomplished. This pioneering method does it through education, correct breathing, relaxation techniques, and exercises.

After practicing obstetrics for forty years, Dr. Dick-Read declared, "Parents—pay attention to childbirth. It is the best investment for a happy, proud and successful life and it is available to poor and rich alike. It pays dividends more valuable than anything money can buy."[1]

Basis for the Dick-Read Techniques

The Dick-Read preparation is based on working with body forces and feelings, and trusting the body to tell you how to respond. For this you must know how to read the signals of childbirth. At the same time, passive relaxation has great importance. Dr. Dick-Read suggests, "The ability to relax during a normal uterine contraction is a basic principle in natural childbirth. Practice and learn complete muscular relaxation as if the ease of your childbirth experience depends on it, because it does!"

Another fundamental of the Dick-Read techniques is emotional support offered by your husband, nurses, and doctor during the time of pregnancy, labor, and delivery. As prospective parents a couple may have heard exaggerated stories about the hostility of hospital personnel toward the desires of the woman in labor. The Dick-Read philosophy requests that both of you verbalize your goals to the health professionals involved. Voice any fears. Let them answer your questions. Make an attempt at rational, objective reasoning even at this time of emotional stress. They will listen and assist you to achieve what you want.

Dick-Read classes teach you—the mother-to-be—to turn inward. You will be able to visualize what is taking place inside you. This turning inward is a difference from some other prepared childbearing methods. It is akin to the meditative technique of yoga, in fact, or perhaps the autosuggestion method of hypnosis. You will be able to make the comparison when you read Chapters 11 or 13. With eyes closed, you may drowse in a sleepy fashion, oblivious to external forces but ready to participate with the actions of nature occurring within. Total concentration is on yourself. Using the breathing and relaxation you have been taught, you will be able to meet each contraction as it comes, but with active control of your response.

Also learned in the Dick-Read preparation classes is how to apply shallow and rapid breathing as the contractions increase in intensity. Panting breathing is the technique employed to prevent pushing prematurely at the start of the second stage of labor and during the delivery. "As the contraction fades," wrote Dr. Dick-Read, "she will relax sleepily, first taking two deep in and out breaths, then quietly resting until the next effort begins. Her drowsiness may be so deep that her mind is concentrated only on the one task of producing her child.

"Just before the head can be seen some women have a strong desire to 'escape' the impending birth," he continued. "When this occurs the woman should remember to ignore the feeling and push firmly for the next two or at the most three contractions. Such concentrated expulsive efforts to help the contraction will quickly overcome the temporary discomfort and desire to escape. Shortly after that the hair on the baby's head will show at the outlet."[2]

Such is the basis for practice of the techniques developed by Dr. Grantly Dick-Read. His fundamental teachings have been modified or expanded and form the foundations for other popular methods of childbirth. We shall describe those methods in the three chapters to follow this one.

Content of the Dick-Read Course

While it is not our intent to present the entire Dick-Read course on these pages, we will give the overall content of this particular approach to childbearing. First we must tell you what Dr. Dick-Read's natural childbirth techniques do *not* offer. They do not offer:

- A pain-free labor and delivery
- A total freedom from anesthesia and other drugs
- Performance without the services of health professionals
- The feeling of failure if you do not come through entirely naturally

What the Dick-Read method *does* offer is:

- Techniques of self-suggestion and mind and body conditioning against discomfort

- The presence and encouragement of your husband as coach during the labor and delivery
- Complete information about what is happening inside your body
- Assistance and furtherance of the forces of nature
- A kind of "psychophysical" support from those attending you in labor

In classes, the Dick-Read school advocates *abdominal breathing*, and instruction is given for a variety of breathing exercises. Some other methods for childbearing prefer chest breathing instead. Typical of the several preparatory respiratory exercises is the one that follows: Stand with feet apart, hands at sides, palms front and raise the hands to shoulder level. Rise on the toes. Complete the movement during deep inhalation and slowly resume starting position with expiration. Repeat six times for practice.

The above type of prenatal practice for lung expansion translates itself finally into learning to pant short breaths, quickly. Thirty-five or forty pants a minute are encouraged, especially during the second stage of labor and just as your baby is being born. Panting enables the head to emerge slowly without extra force needed. You do not bear down. This significantly reduces birth trauma to the baby and avoids excessive pressure on the birth canal.

Episiotomy is the surgical incision of the vulva to prevent laceration at the time of delivery. It is commonly carried out in the practice of American obstetrics. Tearing of the perineum is avoided through proper training in panting, and therefore you may not require an episiotomy.

Accompanying the breathing exercises is *autosuggestion conditioning* which helps you to overcome fear and pain. It is a form of mind control. Actual physical techniques of relaxation are made use of for purposes of this self-conditioning.

Several positions for labor and various physical exercises are taught in Grantly Dick-Read classes.

Figure 14 shows a woman on hands and knees; this position is useful for an exercise of relaxation similar to the Kegel exercises. All the body's muscles are relaxed at once by screwing up the facial muscles, contracting anal and vaginal passages, tightening the buttocks, holding the breath, and then releasing and letting your whole body relax.

Figure 15 shows the woman assuming a squatting position. This is a conditioner for the eventual second stage of labor.

Figure 16 is also a second-stage conditioning exercise. The weight is borne on the back and the legs are held apart with the hands pressing the knees ever wider apart. You can see the action at the opening of the birth canal in this position without using an overhead

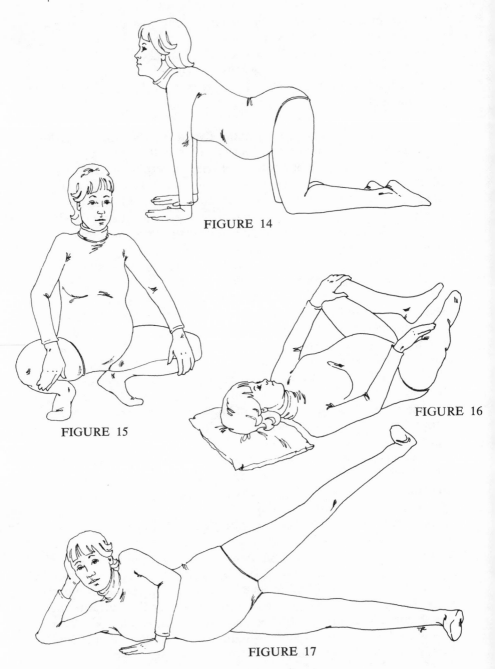

FIGURE 14

FIGURE 15

FIGURE 16

FIGURE 17

mirror. It is an excellent technique for use in home delivery, for it makes the size of the pelvic outlet biggest, and the muscles necessary for pushing are free to work hardest.

Figure 17 shows a muscle strengthening exercise for the adductors. Stretched adductor muscles enlarge the pelvic diameter for creating the widest opening. In this drawing, the woman is raising her leg as high as possible.

Preparation for birth also includes a full *description of the anatomy and physiology* of the process itself. You learn about your body and its functioning and how it develops the body and mind of the child. Diagrams and models are used to illustrate the cervix, vagina, glands, and other body parts concerned with birth. The stages of labor are fully discussed so that you have a full understanding of the process. You will become a thoroughly trained person in childbirth, as will your husband, if he accompanies you. The husband as coach is not mandatory, however, and you may attend classes in the Dick-Read method without him.

For information related to participating in classes for the Dick-Read approach, write to The Natural Childbirth Trust of Great Britain, 26, Seymour Street, London, W.I. England. The trust will tell you where the Dick-Read course may be found.

Variations and Similarities of Childbirth Methods

Preparation courses and written advice on the subject of prepared childbirth share the paradox of being quite dissimilar and yet all the same. They vary in titles such as Dick-Read's Approach, the Lamaze Method, the Psychoprophylaxis, Erna Wright's New Childbirth, Bradley's Husband-Coaching, or the practical lessons suggested by Elisabeth Bing. Each procedure has its somewhat different twist, and yet they come together for the same result, a happy and healthy mother and child. Their individual techniques overlap and are variations of a similar theme.

Idealism is their common point. Ideally, the mother is not exhausted by her ordeal. She feels a tremendous elation from giving birth naturally and actively. An overwhelming sense of love overcomes her as she snuggles the newborn in her arms and immediately feeds him from her breast. She loves her husband more than ever and feels a sense of gratitude to the health professionals who have assisted. After the successful birth, even immediately thereafter, hardly is there a woman who feels she has suffered. Most of the time the mother will plan her next visit for obstetrical care with glee. Of course the father grows a little pale with the idea.[3]

Relationships with Nurses and Doctor Using
the Dick-Read Method

One problem that frequently confronts a woman giving birth under the aegis of personnel practicing the Grantly Dick-Read approach is the unhappiness of other untrained women in labor. One woman progressing comfortably in the Dick-Read method, well toward the second stage, heard the loud cries and moans of a woman in labor from a neighboring room. Concerned, she asked her own obstetrician, "How unnecessary it is that she should suffer. Can't you go and help?"

It was, of course, no business of this obstetrician, and he said so. The cries were not of suffering, he told her, but of fear, and under the influence of narcotic drugs. A perfectly competent doctor was attending her.

After an unhappy hour passed with continuation of the cries, the patient practicing the Dick-Read approach, which she had learned well, proceeded quietly, saying, "I am not having any pain, why should she?" Sometime later her baby was born with no trouble.[4]

Awareness of the emotional needs of women in labor had been growing over the years. Doctors in a few communities, particularly in Florida and Canada, for a long time had thought all of their patients should receive emotional support in labor, and so made this service available by hiring their own nurses. Then some years ago when Grantly Dick-Read was invited to this country to describe his program of prepared childbirth, which he called "natural childbirth," the concept of professionals trained to give support took hold.[5]

In fact, all persons who come in contact with the parturient woman (the woman in the throes of childbirth) should be aware of her preparation and be able to give her support. Even the attendant who might greet the woman in labor when she enters the hospital in the middle of the night can give her an encouraging word, rather than asking, "How bad are the pains, dearie?"

If all are aware of your preparation for childbearing, an immediate rapport will be established among you. They will encourage you with statements such as: "You are doing just fine." "You handled that contraction just beautifully." "It may seem that nothing is progressing now, but it surely looks as if you will take some big steps soon." Most nurses will help you to apply, correct, or modify the breathing and relaxation techniques and be on the lookout for the parts of the body that are tense.

The hospital people will enjoy your company as an alert, active patient who is enjoying her work and achieving the goal—a comfortable, unmedicated birth. The nurses may be able to pick up pointers of support from you that could be applicable to their other patients. Of course, on a rare occasion some nurses are not so helpful or tolerant and that is when you must make use of everything you have learned in preparation to have your baby.

Clarissa Collins Has Her Baby by the Dick-Read Approach

"At five A.M. on the twentieth of last month I awoke to go to the bathroom and just as I stepped out of bed my water broke. My husband was away on a business trip and was not expected back for a week. We knew that I was near my time of labor, and we discussed whether or not he should travel. He said he would not. But I recognized that his manufacturing company was desperate for the sales his trip would bring, and I insisted that he go. Secretly, I felt uneasy about being alone except that I had received valuable instruction from my course in the Grantly Dick-Read approach to natural childbirth. My instructor was there if I needed her, as well as my doctor. And my mother lived only three blocks away.

"When the bag of waters broke I telephoned my obstetrician: 'Hello, Dr. Keller? This is Clarissa Collins. I think my membranes have broken because fluid is leaking down my legs! . . . No, contractions have not started as yet. . . . Oh, they'll start soon? O.K., I'll call my mother and she will drive me to the hospital. Thank you, Doctor. I'll see you there!'

"I experienced a few mild contractions when Mother picked me up and drove me to the hospital door. The nurses prepared me with an enema and a shave. That was the hospital's policy and I didn't have any choice in the matter. The one thing I didn't like at all is that they wouldn't let me up to use the toilet facilities. They insisted I use a bedpan—kind of archaic if you ask me. But I was in no position to argue. My husband might have been my consumer advocate if he had been there. And my mother wasn't trained to be my labor coach. She said, 'Do what the authorities tell you to do, dear. They know and you don't!' I didn't agree but I did what I was told.

"Anyway, things got moving about eight thirty A.M. when the contractions were five minutes apart but easily controllable. By eleven A.M. the nurses moved me into the labor room. Contractions were coming in intervals of four minutes—two minutes—four minutes—two minutes, and so on. I remained in control of the situation as long as I wasn't interfered with. Unfortunately, the nurses were knowledgeable in a childbirth method different from the Dick-Read approach. They wanted me to breathe in a way other than how I was trained. When they insisted, I panicked and lost control. So they backed off! Then I regained my senses and resumed my own method. When I felt the need to pant, I did—when the nurses didn't try to stop me.

"My problem with the nurses ended with my doctor's arrival. He took over and explained to them what my particular method of giving birth was. The Dick-Read approach is not as popular in my city as some others. In fact, very few Dick-Read classes are given in the United States. It was the first natural childbirth method taught in this country and now it's among the rarest.

"Dr. Keller examined me and suddenly discovered that I was fully effaced and almost fully dilated. By the time his orders to wheel me into the delivery room were carried out, I was panting and blowing to keep from pushing. I felt the baby was ready to come. Following his sterile scrub, my obstetrician said we were all set to proceed with the birthing. 'You can push,' he told me. That was welcome news!

"I pushed when he said to push, panted when he said to pant, and then there was my baby's head. It was the most fantastic, rewarding, wonderful sight. What a thrilling experience to see a live, wiggling creature coming out of my body. I can't thank my Dick-Read instructor and Dr. Keller enough for making it so easy for me. I didn't need an episiotomy and walked back to my room within forty minutes after cuddling my little one for a half hour. Both of us went home, my daughter and I, in just two days, and my husband flew home that same day, too."

NOTES FOR CHAPTER SEVEN

1. Grantly Dick-Read, *The Natural Childbirth Primer* (New York: Harper & Row, 1956).

2. Grantly Dick-Read, *Childbirth Without Fear* (New York: Harper & Row, 1952).

3. Florence E. Hoff, "Natural Childbirth: How Any Nurse Can Help," *American Journal of Nursing* 69:1451–53 (July 1969).

4. Dick-Read, *Childbirth Without Fear.*

5. Flora Hommel, "Natural Childbirth—Nurses in Private Practice as Monitrices," *American Journal of Nursing* 69:1447–50 (July 1969).

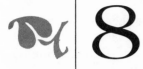

8

The Lamaze Method

At this moment I look upon my husband and child and thank you for giving us the opportunity of being together as a threesome immediately upon the arrival of Polly. Giving birth to Polly was, quite honestly, the hardest work I've ever experienced. Yet, I feel I've accomplished something so rewarding and spectacular that I'm still shocked at my own strength. Kevin and I say "Thank you, Mrs. Yoffe" for giving us the tools to completely share our love in the birth of our child.
—MARILYN PORTER O'HAGIN, 1977

The Log of the Arrival of Jules Walker

At 12:55 A.M.: I awoke to the sound of Joan's cleansing inhalation. It was one of the breathing exercises we had learned while attending classes together in the Lamaze method of childbirth. We had prepared ourselves for this moment. My wife was having labor contractions. They were twenty-five seconds long and coming at one-minute intervals.

1:30 A.M.: Joan insisted on putting a load of laundry into the washing machine. I went to the basement to assist her.

2:00 A.M.: She felt slightly stronger contractions which lasted forty-five seconds at two- to three-minute intervals. We discussed telephoning Bernice Yoffe, R.N., our instructor in the Lamaze method, but we agreed that she should be allowed to sleep a little longer. Bernice was our "monitrice" who would be in attendance with advice and encouragement during labor and delivery.

2:40 A.M.: Joan felt the need to breathe using the slow chest technique, since her contractions were stronger. We returned to bed and tried to sleep, but dozing left her unprepared for more contractions. I felt Joan's abdomen move upward and become hard like a board as labor's forceful movements passed through her uterus. We stayed awake so that she could remain in control of each contraction.

3:20 A.M.: We walked to the kitchen where I ate breakfast. Joan ate nothing. We had been taught that now was a time when she should have an empty stomach.

4:50 A.M.: We moved the washed clothes to the dryer and put another bundle into the washing machine. It was the last job Joan wished to do before going to the hospital. Her valise had been packed for weeks. Her contractions were now irregular—some five minutes apart and each lasting two minutes—alternately strong and mild.

5:20 A.M.: The bag of waters broke, and Joan was saturated with amniotic fluid tinged with blood. She changed her clothing. I telephoned the doctor and Bernice to say that we were heading for the hospital.

5:45 A.M.: It was cold and dark on this first morning in January. Some late-hour revelers were on the way home from their New Year's celebration. My wife was smiling, feeling cheerful and enthusiastic with the advent of our new baby. She made me feel that way, too.

5:55 A.M.: I went with Joan to the maternity floor, then walked to the hospital admitting office and filled in the necessary papers. Our obstetrician arrived. He said he would call me into the labor room after my wife had her enema.

6:40 A.M.: As I stood outside the door of the labor room, Bernice Yoffe arrived. She went into the room speaking words of encouragement.

7:15 A.M.: I assisted Joan with a back massage and timed the contractions. The physician entered to examine my wife.

8:00 A.M.: Her cervical dilation came faster now. Joan was breathing with the rhythmic panting technique and used occasional blowing because her contractions were really severe. I helped to coach her in the breathing technique. Bernice did also. Joan felt the compulsion to push, but blowing prevented premature pushing. I counted the contraction seconds for her and kept the rhythm of breathing. Bernice encouraged us with assurances that everything was normal.

8:40 A.M.: The doctor told Joan that she may now bear down and ordered the nurse to wheel her to the delivery room.

8:45 A.M.: In the doctors' dressing room, I donned a green scrub suit, cap, mask, and cloth shoes while our obstetrician scrubbed for the procedure.

8:52 A.M.: After injecting a local anesthetic into her perineum, the physician performed an episiotomy. He asked Joan to hold back from pushing. Bernice adjusted the mirror above the delivery table so that Joan and I could view the proceedings.

The bright morning sun reflected off the instruments and other gleaming equipment. The room was large, bright, and airy. Use of artificial light was unnecessary.

9:09 A.M.: Joan asked to be allowed to bear down, and the physician agreed. She knew that each push made her birth canal open wider. She smiled with joy even in hard labor. Bernice's instructions had been to bear down with a deep breath, lips pursed, chin forward, pushing forward. I reminded Joan of the instructions. We cheered her on.

9:21 A.M.: The dark hair on our newborn's head came into view. We saw it in the mirror. With another contraction the opening got wider.

9:26 A.M.: Our baby slid out face down, head conical. It turned, and I saw the eyes, nose, ears, and mouth. The newborn was smiling. With a sheet between his hands, the doctor grasped the head at the next contraction and pulled. A shoulder popped out, then another, and the rest of the body came. He caught the infant, placed it on Joan's abdomen, and we saw it was a boy. I lifted my wife's shoulders for her to get a closer view of our baby.

9:30 A.M.: Our son, Jules Louis Walker, gave a little cry and then a louder one. The obstetrical nurse moved to Joan's side, prepared to suction away mucus from the child's eyes, nose, and mouth. The doctor clamped the cord, cut it, and put Jules in a padded metal cradle off to the side. I asked the nurse to make the baby cry again so that he would pull in more air. She tapped his feet. He took a breath, cried loudly, and grew pinker in color. She gave him a little stimulating oxygen and we heard him cry some more. Joan and I hugged each other. We whispered words of love. This was the most joyous of experiences, precious moments in our lives.

The Lamaze Method of Psychoprophylactic Childbirth

Joan and I had attended classes in the Lamaze Method of Psychoprophylactic Childbirth in our instructor's home. As mentioned, Bernice Yoffe was also Joan's monitrice during her hours in labor and delivery. The monitrice is a support person who teaches the couple how to confront childbirth. She may or may not accompany them all

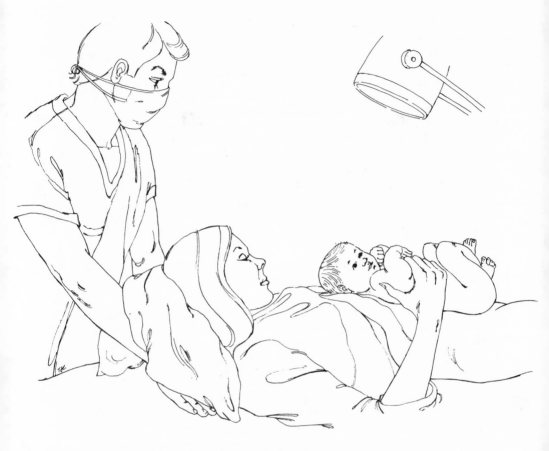

FIGURE 18

the way through the childbearing process. The concept of having a monitrice was one of the many procedures devised by Fernand Lamaze and his assistant, Pierre Vellay—the two physicians who introduced psychoprophylaxis in France. From there the method's procedures have spread all over the world.

Psychoprophylactic childbirth was endorsed in 1956 by Pope Pius XII as a "benefit for the mother" which "fully conforms to the will of the Creator." The pope said, "Science therefore may utilize the findings of experimental psychology, physiology and gynecology, as is being done by the psychoprophylactic method, in order to eliminate the causes for mistakes and to remove the pain-producing conditioned reflexes, so that birth can become as painless as possible. The holy scripture does not forbid this."

As we mentioned in Chapter 1, psychoprophylaxis is based on the work of Russian practitioners, especially the psychological investigations of the Pavlovian school into conditioned reflexes. It teaches women how to counteract to the pain of labor by enlightening them. Husbands and mothers-to-be also learn about sexual anatomy, the functions and development of body organs, the chemistry of glands and hormones, the biology of reproduction and conception, and the psychology of pregnancy, including its effects on both people in a couple relationship.

The Lamaze method goes much further than the Dick-Read Approach. There are detailed discussions of sex and reproduction, focusing on them as irreversible products of evolution and the natural laws of survival and putting aside their social and moral aspects. All aspects of maternity are included in the discussions: emotional preparation, physical changes, fetal development, proper diet, conditioning exercises, necessary breathing, muscle control for labor, the father's role, and the actual birth process.

Varying from the Dick-Read approach still further, Lamaze preparation offers an active, directive psychological analgesia to modify the perception of pain. Usually, no drugs are taken. Instead, this psychological direction gives the woman something to do besides tense her muscles. Because you are using a higher level of conscious activity, controlled breathing, and letting go of uninvolved muscles, an "automatic response" takes over. It is a process of turning outward, as opposed to the inward focus of the Dick-Read method.

The husband or friend in whom the pregnant woman has confidence takes training with her. He acts as her coach and assists with conditioning her reflexes to respond. By the husband putting the pressure on the inner thigh muscle of his wife's leg, for instance, he creates an artificial stimulus long before labor. The pressure is to build up this conditioned or automatic response. She goes into her relaxation and breathing techniques—a form of psychological analgesia.

The Key Is the Total Change in Attitude

The American birth rate is up from a 1976 low. Approximately 3.4 million babies were born in 1977, or about 200,000 more than had been expected. Experts are not very surprised. The American birth rate has elevated because the number of women in the childbearing ages of fifteen to forty-four is swollen with the ranks of girls born during the baby boom after World War II. They are now passing through their prime years of fertility. Actually, it is surprising that the

108 |

birth rate has remained so low for so long. Many experts have long anticipated an "echo" effect of the postwar baby boom.[1]

A fair slice of this population explosion has been born via the psychoprophylactic method of Dr. Lamaze. A change in attitude for women is the reason. A minor alteration in emphasis has made child-bearing a positive experience rather than one filled with pain and fear. The experiences of mothers with the Lamaze method have been so rewarding they have become almost messianic about spreading its practice. In fact, the prepared childbirth experience has extended to China. Having a baby this way was even endorsed by the late Chair-man Mao. Also all French women must by law be given a chance to practice *La Methode*. And we have already told you of its endorse-ment by the Soviet Government and the pope.

Psychoprophylaxis aims to take this changed attitude of women and recondition it to the positive belief that having babies is not only a joy, but can be easier if they stay in control of their bodies and the birth at all times. It has the mother deliver the baby *to* the doctor or nurse-midwife herself, in place of the nonparticipating approach where she was delivered *of* her baby by the health professional attending her.

Our last statement is not semantics. This changed attitude trans-forms childbirth from an ordeal to an ecstatic experience in 90 per-cent of cases. The key is a deemphasis of pain and a fuller control of your body. There is comfort even with having contractions. The Lamaze instruction is: "Think of each contraction as a wave at the seaside, rising to a peak, breaking, and then running out again over the sand. It can be a great deal of fun to ride through these large waves if you dive through with absolute control of your body and your breathing."

Richard S. Banfield, Jr., M.D., describes active participation in the birth of your child in another way. The obstetrician says: "Childbirth has been compared to climbing a mountain. Who would think of getting medication as the ascent began and then being anesthetized just short of the peak—being carried to the pinnacle, brought down, awakened, and told you have been to the top. The Lamaze method enables you to go to the top, take in all the beauty of that unforget-table moment of delivery."

Physical and Psychological Preparation Through Classes

During the last two months of pregnancy, Joan and I had enrolled in training classes taught by Mrs. Yoffe, who is one of many hundreds of accredited instructors in the Lamaze method. They teach in every corner of the United States and parts of Canada. Classes are available for women alone if their mates are not able to attend, but the vast majority of men do come. As mentioned before the man's role is an active and important one; he supports his mate physically and psychologically during training and in actual labor and delivery, making childbearing a total family experience. The classes run about two hours each and start at the end of the seventh month of pregnancy.

The *first class* furnishes a full orientation of what the five or six weekly sessions are about. In the first class one learns the different phases of childbirth. Additional areas of instruction include how to cooperate with normal muscular contractions, the response to obstetrical guidance, and the husband as helper or coach.

At the *second class, The Birth Atlas*, which is a series of photographs showing plaster models of the fetus created by the Maternity Center Association, is used to illustrate what actually happens inside the uterus. The discomforts of pregnancy are discussed, and couples have a chance to have their questions answered. An instructor will demonstrate the exercises of concentration-relaxation, the response to commands to tense or relax an arm or a leg, and the procedure for conditioned reflexes when needed. The instructor shows correct posture and body building for the effort of labor. The exercises are fun and uplifting. Couples often become friends with each other and share experiences.

For the *third session* all is reviewed quickly and new breathing exercises are added. The deep cleansing breath announces the coming of a contraction; the slow chest breathing, in through the nose and out through the mouth, is reserved for the beginning stage of labor; the shallow and quick panting is used at the second stage; the panting-blowing breaths are employed at the end of the second stage. Slow chest breathing or the panting are used at a woman's discretion, depending on the strength of contractions. Diagrams shown in the class depict how each contraction shortens, thins, and flattens the cervix during the three stages of labor.

The *fourth class* is a review of everything learned to that point. Classmates demonstrate their exercises and the instructor/monitrice corrects any errors. The couples listen to a recording of an actual labor and delivery which helps them picture themselves in the delivery room. The effects of anesthesia and other drugs on the mother and child are discussed. And finally, the instructor demonstrates the position and techniques for bearing down during expulsion of the baby.

The *fifth class* includes slides of the actual delivery of a baby using the Lamaze method. More remarkable even than the sight of the infant leaving the birth canal is the ecstatic expression on the face of the mother as she watches her newborn coming into the world. Another recording played reviews all the exercises learned.

A possible *sixth class* is the showing of a color film with all the sights and sounds of a woman giving birth to a healthy baby by the psychoprophylactic procedure. The couples are taken through each technique with its application at the appropriate time. Then the instructor lectures on postpartum, parenting, infant behavior, and breast feeding. The couples ask questions. They end with feeling quite prepared for the blessed event to come.

The fee for the Lamaze course depends on geographic location but ranges from $25 to $75 per couple. For information about the location nearest to you, write to the American Society for Psycho-Prophylaxis in Obstetrics, Inc., Box 725, Midtown Station, New York, New York, 10018.

"Thank You, Dr. Lamaze"

Dr. Fernand Lamaze wrote a book published in France in 1956 about his work carried out at the Maternite' du Me'tallurgiste. It was translated and published in the English language in Great Britain in 1958, but the psychoprophylactic method of "painless childbirth" did not really become popular in the United States until Marjorie Karmel wrote her book.

We began this chapter with a quote from Marilyn Porter O'Hagin's letter to Nurse Yoffe where she wrote "Thank you, Mrs. Yoffe." Ms. O'Hagin is actually referring to the Karmel book, *Thank You, Dr. Lamaze*. Published in 1959, Marjorie Karmel dedicated her writing effort to the memory of Dr. Lamaze and his modification of Pavlov's original contribution to painless childbirth. The work of Fernand Lamaze has been carried on by his friend and fellow practitioner, Dr. Pierre Vellay, who has published his own book called *Childbirth with Confidence*.

Indeed, a number of variations of the Lamaze method have evolved since Dr. Lamaze brought back ideas for his techniques from his first trip to Leningrad in 1952. The next chapter will briefly describe those variations.

NOTES FOR CHAPTER EIGHT

1. Robert Reinhold, "Birth Rate Is Rising from 1976 Low," *The New York Times,* July 24, 1977.

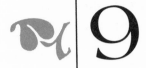

9

Further Development of the Lamaze Method

During the first weeks, I used to lie long hours with the baby in my arms, watching her asleep; sometimes catching a gaze from her eyes; feeling very near the edge, the mystery, perhaps the knowledge of life. This soul in the newly created body which answered my gaze with such apparently old eyes—the eyes of Eternity—gazing into mine with love. Love, perhaps, was the answer of all. What words could describe this joy? What wonder that I, who am a writer, cannot find any words at all!
—ISADORA DUNCAN, *My Life*

The Spreading Popularity of Psychoprophylaxis

As time passes, more and more couples are participating in the natural delivery of their children. The Lamaze method is the most popular of the natural techniques among Americans. Use of it is spreading, and some supporters have developed further variations. Innovators have brought about new benefits of psychoprophylaxis by altering the original techniques.

There are many modernizers of the psychoprophylactic prepared childbirth approach. Chief among its exponents but with their own variations are Elisabeth Bing, Erna Wright, and Sheila Kitzinger. Dr. Vellay, and his student in independent practice, Ingrid Mitchell, have made their changes as well.

Services Offered by Elisabeth Bing

Elisabeth Bing, a trained physical therapist, seems to be *the* authority on the Lamaze method of prepared childbirth and other maternity matters in the United States. She is clinical assistant professor for the Department of Obstetrics-Gynecology at New York Medical College. Mrs. Bing offers her know-how in classes held at The Elisabeth Bing Center for Parents, 164 West Seventy-ninth Street, New York, New York 10024. She has written several books on pregnancy, labor, and delivery, and postpartum care. Her most recent book is *Making Love During Pregnancy.* Another useful book by her that explores her variations on the Lamaze method is *Six Practical Lessons for an Easier Childbirth.*

Mrs. Bing is noted for her training of monitrices and nurses in the Lamaze method as well as of pregnant women. Bing-trained assistants play a key role in the team approach to labor. Because of Lamaze nurses, the obstetrician generally need not be called until the patient's active phase of labor.[1]

At the Bing Center the mother-to-be and her spouse are given a six-week course of ninety-minute segments to prepare them for the big event. This course is taken at the end of the seventh month of pregnancy. Couples learn the how, what, and when of delivery; women are taught exercises that emphasize the relaxation and breathing techniques common to the psychoprophylactic method. Mrs. Bing charges $75 and limits her classes to ten couples per session.[2]

Her assistants also teach the women relaxation techniques, breath control, and abdominal-, back-, and pelvic-strengthening exercises that are set to music. It is actually a series of dance procedures. The sessions are not limited to those who intend to employ Lamaze techniques exclusively. Payment of $25 buys five one-hour dance sessions.

The Elisabeth Bing Center for Parents additionally offers postpartum exercises. These are dance movements designated as a "re-education" of the abdominal muscles after delivery to get new mothers back to prepregnancy svelteness. Five one-hour sessions are offered at a fee of $25.

There are now variations on the Bing methods. Some of Mrs. Bing's disciples have broken away and formed their own groups. But in lecturing to nurses and others, this expert in psychoprophylaxis says herself: "You do have to change with the times. Childbirth methods will vary with what works most effectively. Nothing is static!"

Changes Preferred by Elisabeth Bing

Under the Lamaze techniques three or four forms of breathing are taught. This is the first area where Mrs. Bing changes the normal pattern. Rather than simple exhalation through the mouth as suggested by Lamaze, the Bing technique is to produce a whistling sound during exhaling. She believes that this sound will help to keep a good rhythm. Also Bing says there is no arbitrary cutoff point for moving from the first to the second level of breathing, since your state of relaxation during the quiet breathing period determines which level you maintain. She recommends that you change breathing levels by tapping out a ¼ rhythm on your thigh. You can even sing a ¼ rhythm tune.

In the second stage of labor, the pushing stage, Bing does not want you to put your chin on the chest while bearing down. If you do, she says, the escape of air will be prevented. Tilt the head forward, suggests Mrs. Bing, so as to avoid increased blood circulation to the face by letting air release. This differs from the original Lamaze method.

The Lamaze and Bing schools do not differ when it comes to relaxation exercises and physical conditioning exercises. They combine physical drills with appropriate breathing. A woman learns the pelvic rock, the Kegel exercise, the pelvic floor contraction, the tailor exercise, and other physical conditionings. We shall be describing these exercises. Neuromuscular control is achieved under the Bing variation by tensing one side of the body and leaving the other side limp. Thus, when the uterus contracts, the rest of the body will be made to relax.

Further Variations by Erna Wright

Also an exponent of the Lamaze method rather than of the Dick-Read approach, Erna Wright, an Englishwoman, is a nurse-midwife, who has conducted many deliveries. Her book, *The New Childbirth*, has been approved by the American Society for Psychoprophylaxis in Obstetrics, Inc. (ASPO). Mrs. Wright's variations on the Lamaze techniques are further described in that book.

The breathing procedure taught in the Wright school calls for the use of the rib muscles to cause a higher-than-normal chest breathing.

She calls it "intercostal breathing," which is applied by the mother-to-be when she nears "level B." This B level is reached, says Mrs. Wright, by having the ribs swing out with each inhaling breath. She suggests that a woman change breathing levels during single contractions to achieve distraction from discomfort. Mouth the word "out," says this nurse-midwife-author, in order to keep the cheeks taut during exhaling.

While most Lamaze instructors teach what they call dissociation drills or neuromuscular exercises that have you perform a series of muscular control exercises to contract and relax opposite muscles, Mrs. Wright differs. She wants no artificial contractions and relaxations of these opposite sides or separate muscles. Her simple rule is to tense your muscles during inhalation and relax them during exhalation. Using her easy technique, there is not so much to think about while in the throes of a contraction.

Erna Wright, R.N., holds essentially to the same techniques as does Dr. Lamaze when it comes to the physical conditioning and other comfort measures taught in classes.

Sheila Kitzinger Makes Some Lamaze Alterations

In two of her books, *The Experience of Childbirth* and *Giving Birth*, Sheila Kitzinger, a childbirth educator, indicates she has made some alterations in the Lamaze method that she teaches in classes. The Kitzinger techniques include a form of mouth-centered breathing that she calls "hummingbird" breathing. You feel it almost exclusively in the mouth. It starts above the breastbone and advances in split seconds away from the level of the throat so as to avoid catching the breath in the throat. It is a very gentle and soft form of breathing.

The Kitzinger school also differs from the pure psychoprophylactic method when the baby glides down the birth canal. Then Sheila Kitzinger advises an easy and gentle pushing effort by the mother. This is especially recommended for the mother who has given birth before.

Her other variation for the second stage is to push with your abdomen relaxed instead of with contracted abdominal muscles. Kitzinger says that contracted abdominal muscles cause the birth canal to stay tight and narrow. Her directions are to open the mouth slightly by smiling. This will relax the abdomen. It is quite a different procedure than what is taught for the expulsion of the baby in the original Lamaze classes.

To achieve neuromuscular control and physical conditioning, this childbirth educator suggests some variations, too. Her pelvic rocking

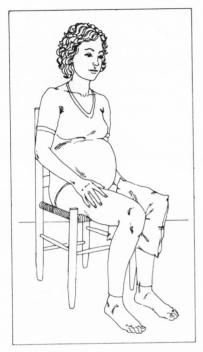

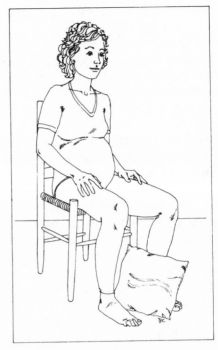

FIGURE 19   FIGURE 20

exercise differs. Lamaze teaches you to rock your pelvis standing up, but Kitzinger suggests that by resting on all fours, with your back arched like a cat, you can involve the shoulders in the motion of your pelvis for more effective conditioning.

The Kegel exercise for reducing pregnancy discomfort from pelvic congestion is accomplished by contracting the muscles around the vagina as if you were trying to stop or hold from urinating. During labor, the pressure is on the pelvic floor and the opening needs to be relaxed in order to let the baby out of the birth canal. This will be achieved more readily if you learn to control these muscles.

A good technique for practicing is shown. Sit in a chair with feet flat on the floor and a pillow held tightly between the knees (Figure 19). Contract the vaginal muscles, hold tight for a few seconds and slowly release them until the pillow falls to the floor (Figure 20).

Sheila Kitzinger carries this exercise further by requiring that the alternate contractions and relaxations include the gluteal muscles in the buttocks. After delivery, continuing with the Kegel exercises will one up and firm the whole area so as to tighten the vaginal vault.

Pierre Vellay Adds His Variations

Pierre Vellay, M.D., who is secretary of the International Society for Psychoprophylaxis in Obstetrics in Paris, France, learned the psychoprophylactic method from Dr. Fernand Lamaze. Already an elderly man when he brought the Pavlovian techniques to his metal worker's clinic, Dr. Lamaze taught many colleagues. Dr. Vellay was among them. When the master died of heart disease in 1957, the psychoprophylactic method did not die with him. His students carried on the work.

Dr. Vellay's current base of operation is the Clinique du Belvedere in Paris from where he disseminates information about the Lamaze method. He has written three books, *Childbirth Without Pain, Sex Development and Maternity*, and *Childbirth with Confidence*. In them, it is apparent that Dr. Vellay is steadily evolving his own method away from the original form taught by Dr. Lamaze.

Dr. Vellay has modified the breathing techniques slightly by suggesting that breathing should be audible. Like Elisabeth Bing, he says the sound could be one of whistling or "whooshing." Also he eliminates any of the characteristics of panting.

Dr. Vellay has expanded the tailor exercise somewhat. The *tailor exercise* (Figure 21) is a physical conditioning technique where the woman sits cross-legged on a hard surface, her back straight but slightly rounded to avoid back strain. The coach, who may be her husband, places his hands on the outside of her thighs. Against the pressure of his hands, the woman attempts to hold open her thighs. The modification of this exercise by Dr. Vellay involves separating the knees and bringing the soles together.

The tailor exercise, including Dr. Vellay's variation, stretches your body and relaxes the pelvic floor so that the baby may pass through the birth canal with more ease.

Another way to accomplish the tailor exercise is on the back. Dr. Vellay does not use this technique but the other innovators do. While lying on the floor, the knees are raised and moved outward as the soles come together. You readily move the walls of the vagina away from each other this way.

Ingrid Mitchell Holds to the Vellay Technique

Trained as a monitrice by Pierre Vellay in Paris during the winter of 1964–65, Ingrid Mitchell has been teaching the psychoprophylactic method in the United States as an accredited member of ASPO.

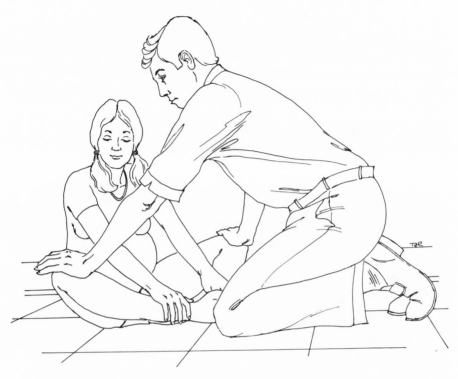

FIGURE 21

She is a registered midwife. Mrs. Mitchell and Mrs. Bing have worked together on numerous occasions to further the Lamaze method of childbirth, but they differ a little in their approach.

The book written by Ingrid Mitchell, *Giving Birth Together*, indicates no great variation from the original Lamaze technique. She has retained almost all of it. However, Mrs. Mitchell has affiliated herself closely with the teachings of Dr. Vellay, and there is hardly any difference between her techniques and his. One innovation of her own, which has altered his application of the tailor exercise, is that she has her clients perform it on their backs as do the other innovators.

"Knock 'Em Out, Drag 'Em Out" Is Not Acceptable

Perhaps you have noticed that the techniques of natural childbirth are growing more popular with time. This has happened because more doctors and nurses are getting involved. Greater understanding and wider acceptance are occurring. The benefits of psychoprophylaxis are being fully acknowledged at last and support is coming from formerly conservative exponents of the use of technology in childbirth. Why? Mostly because they see the excellent results. And the medical consumer movement, pressed home by women, is a factor as well. "We are not patients," women are saying. "The birth process is perfectly normal and natural; therefore, we want to deliver our babies naturally. Prepare us and we will do that. Prepare our partners and they will help us."

The modern trend is away from the traditional "knock 'em out, drag 'em out" approach, as it has been disdainfully referred to. Expecting couples don't accept that anymore.

NOTES FOR CHAPTER NINE

1. Clement Yahia and Priscilla R. Ulin, "Preliminary Experience with a Psychophysical Program of Preparation for Childbirth," *American Journal of Obstetrics and Gynecology* 93:942–50 (December 1, 1965).

2. Deborah Haber, "Exercise!" *New York* 5:59–60 (October 1977).

10

Bradley Husband-Coached Natural Childbirth

*After twenty-six years and over thirteen thousand
births without a single maternal mortality I am
deeply and sincerely convinced that the constant
presence of a loved and loving husband serves
to foster a state of serenity in the mother's mind
that is comparable to a part of the religious
serenity that has aided some mothers for
centuries to follow their instinctive abilities calmly
and give birth actively to their babies. Your
presence as a trained and loving helper will foster
that serenity in your wife as she becomes a mother.*
—ROBERT A. BRADLEY, M.D.
Husband-Coached Childbirth

The Study Conducted by Dr. Bradley

Robert A. Bradley, M.D., the man who developed the concept of husband-coached natural childbirth, says he would not allow even a stray dog into the delivery room to witness a medicated mother being put to sleep and her even sleepier baby being "delivered."

"The dog would get sick!" explains Dr. Bradley. In 1947, he stumbled upon an excellent innovation in obstetrics—the inclusion of a trained, prepared husband as a participating member of the birth team. The husband's assigned goal is to coach his wife to achieve a spontaneous, unmedicated birth. (Note that we have written "birth" rather than "delivery" because exponents of the Bradley method do not accept that a woman is delivered of her baby. She gives birth to it.)

A study Dr. Bradley conducted using four thousand consecutive cases histories refuted the ancient myths of infections from the presence of "dirty" husbands and "fainting" husbands. All that is needed to prevent infections is to have the men properly gowned, capped, and masked—and none of them faint either!

His study further showed that all stages of labor were shortened; there was a low incidence of forceps application—96.4 percent of the vaginal deliveries were spontaneous birth; both husbands and wives were filled with enthusiasm and joy by their respective roles and the total experience of birth; husbands did not "get in the way" or in any way interfere—rather, as coaches they had a calming and soothing effect on their wives and added a note of good humor. The unmedicated mothers were able to walk back from the delivery room immediately after giving birth, and postpartum hospital stays were phenomenally shortened.

The women, in fact, stayed in the hospital following the birth for an average of only twenty-four hours. Hundreds of the four thousand mothers remained for only the two hours that the hospital required. Essentially, Dr. Bradley's study proved that hospitals are for sick people and postpartum women are not sick.

Today's Consumer in the Medical Marketplace

Just as Americans have become more consumer-conscious in the marketplace, they have become more knowledgeable about the quality of obstetrical care they pay for. Alibis are no longer acceptable. When an obstetrician gives a vague alibi about the husband's violating the sterile delivery room, today's man may retort that having a baby is hardly a surgical operation. Obstetrician Bradley agrees. He promotes the principles of true natural childbirth, including the concept of an active role for the husband as "labor coach." The Bradley method of husband-coached labor and birth has been popularly accepted throughout most of the United States and several areas of Canada.

In 1962, Dr. Bradley prepared a paper based on his study of husbands in the labor and delivery rooms. It was published in the official journal of the Academy of Psychosomatic Medicine (*Psychosomatics* III (6) [1962]). The article was promptly reviewed in international news wire services, newspapers, magazines, etc., and he received a deluge of requests for interviews, lectures, and articles. In four years nearly nine thousand requests for reprints came in from the general public. By then his number of successful births by the husband-coached method had grown to eight thousand. Eventually, Dr. Bradley wrote *Husband-Coached Childbirth,* a book directed to a popular audience.

In the medical marketplace the pregnant consumer has made her demands known. She has joined together with her husband and other dedicated women and formed two organizations: the International Childbirth Education Association and the La Leche League, International. The latter organization is concerned with breast feeding, which is an integral part of the new concept of prepared parenthood. Members of both associations have made their wants known. Their influence has been felt in the United States and many other countries. In addition, the American Academy of Husband-Coached Childbirth has been created. Instructors affiliated with the academy take extensive training and are required to continue their education. For help in locating a Bradley-method instructor near your home or to become an instructor yourself, write to The American Academy of Husband-Coached Childbirth, P.O. Box 5224, Sherman Oaks, California 91413.

The fertile younger generation are shouting their requests. They are taking part in a childbirth rebellion and using the Bradley husband-coaching method as their tool. They plea fervently, "Please, Doctors, we'd rather do it ourselves!" The young potential parents insist that they, the public, are the "customers," and that hospitals and physicians are servants of the public who should cater to their wants or be deprived of their business. A lot of doctors and hospital administrators are listening. Many concur that hospitals are primarily tax-free *public* institutions and secondarily *medical* institutions. The pregnant medical consumer is winning her battle, and the Bradley philosophy is encouraging her to fight.

The Role of the Husband During Labor

The husband's role during his wife's labor is vital, according to the Bradley philosophy. He has a clear-cut right to be with his wife. Incidentally, although the method is called husband-coached childbirth, another partner may be needed or preferred, such as a mother, sister, or a friend. However, the husband is usually the best coach.

In ideal circumstances, the husband must be able both to supervise and support his wife during labor—helping her to maintain total relaxation and providing reassurance. He may have to help her change position, for example, even though she might feel reluctant to move; he may have to remind her of her breathing technique, should she forget. In other words, the husband-coach is no "handholder." He can literally make or break his wife's birth experience.

One account of a natural birth that we have heard describes a nurse's refusal to let the husband stay with his wife while she was being "prepped." By the time he was allowed to rejoin her, the labor pains had become so severe that the wife wanted an injection to relieve them.

Seeing that his wife was on the verge of losing control, he quickly began the Bradley techniques to help her relax. Speaking softly to calm her, applying back pressure when and where needed, giving her ice chips to suck on, and demonstrating to her how to breathe correctly, the husband completely involved himself with helping his wife get through labor.

She regained control. The couple complimented each other upon their mutual cooperation toward a successful natural childbirth.

Margaret Marks Higle, a member of the American Academy of Husband-Coached Childbirth and Connecticut regional director of the Childbirth Education Association of Metropolitan New York, who admits to making modifications in teaching the Bradley method, told us of another incident where a husband became his wife's spokesperson. Ms. Higle said, "A pregnant woman had an agreement with her obstetrician that she would give birth sitting up in the physiological position without straps on the arms or stirrups for the legs. This way she could give birth rather than be delivered.

"The sitting position is physiologically best for her and her baby and more comfortable, less restricting, and not undignified. Unless a woman is medicated for a medical problem, there is no real reason why she must have her legs up in stirrups and her arms strapped down," Ms. Higle explained.

"Well, despite the agreement with her doctor, when the woman's husband left to put on his delivery room greens at the very last minute, the obstetrical nursing staff placed her legs up in stirrups. That is a good example of why the husband should don his delivery room greens far in advance of the delivery. Because she was in the height of labor pushing, this woman let herself be overwhelmed by the hospital staff. When the man returned and asked his wife whether she wanted that position and heard that she did not, he insisted they take her down. He became her persistent spokesperson and made demands. The staff complied."

Very often from the wife's point of view, it is better if her husband leads her through childbirth. She knows and trusts him. By the time the first baby arrives, the woman has probably developed a certain amount of faith in her mate's dependability during times of crises. On the other hand, a woman may not even know the doctor or midwife who delivers her baby because of some emergency or alteration in scheduling the delivery. Her husband's reliable coaching is a primary means for overcoming any possible lack of confidence.

The Bradley Method Encourages Breast Feeding

As we have seen the Bradley method provides studied rules for coaching one's wife through pregnancy, labor, and birth. Bradley has also made recommendations on the man's role in breast-feeding the baby.

Dr. Bradley encourages nursing. At one time he said, "The law of change is manifest in many ways in obstetrics. Alert doctors recognize that they are unaware, unprepared, and inexperienced in the art of breast feeding, and so they encourage experienced breast-feeding mothers to participate in La Leche League (The Milk League) activities and pass their womanly knowledge on to the awkward, frightened, newly pregnant woman. As an obstetrician I know nothing about breast feeding except, selfishly, how it helps to separate placentas spontaneously at birth, reduce the incidence of postpartum hemorrhage, and maintain new mothers without 'tired blood' by postponing menses."[1]

We will fully discuss breast feeding in Chapter 20.

Content of the Bradley Husband-Coached Techniques

We have said that Dr. Bradley started using husbands as coaches after he noticed how his patients could remain calm and relaxed during contractions only when their husbands were by their sides. If the men left the room—even for just a few moments—their wives' labors were adversely affected. Without the husbands, the women immediately became anxious, tense, and unable to relax. As a result, their contractions quickly began to feel painful.

One might wonder what it is that the men do to relax their wives. What is the content of the various Bradley husband-coached techniques?

For starters, the first class in husband-coaching is held early in the pregnancy—at the third month. This session provides much valuable information for women and their spouses. Especially vital is nutritional information in the event the mother-to-be does not have a doctor who advises her. She is told of no-nos in drug use and how to stay comfortable while pregnant. Some simple exercises are given for maintenance of good posture, back comfort, and for getting muscles ready for labor and birth. The husband does these easy exercises with his wife which makes it fun. This togetherness encourages her to keep up with the exercises during the ensuing months of waiting.

Then eight two-hour sessions offer the rest of a highly constructive program of techniques. These sessions are given once a week starting in the sixth or seventh month of pregnancy. They are then followed by review classes every other week until birth. The husband and wife both attend. The fee ranges from $40 to $75, depending on the amount of educational material supplied by the instructor.

In the sessions a man learns that one of his major functions is to observe his mate. He knows better than anyone just how much she can take, since he has seen her when not in pain or sick. In his mind, the husband can make the comparison and alert the medical personnel if all is not well. It is a heavy responsibility.

One man who took the Bradley course, but who was evidentally brought up in a home where childbirth was considered "woman's work," refused to enter the delivery room with his wife. He said he just didn't feel it was his job. He stayed with her in labor and provided much encouragement. Then the nurses wheeled her away. When told he was the father of a healthy baby boy, the man's first remark was, "You know, I felt as if they'd cut off my right arm when they took my wife in and left me out here. Next time I'll surely go into the birthing room with her."

The husband times the contractions, gets his wife little sips of water for mouth washing, moistens her forehead with a cool cloth, rolls the bed up and down as required, helps her turn from one side to the other, carries on diverting conversation between contractions and perhaps tells jokes, plays cards with her, and does other little things for entertainment. He does everything possible to cause time to speed along and make the laboring comfortable. Women repeat over and over that it is really more pleasant to have the husband's familiar face to look at than a nurse who is a stranger.

The man provides the nurses with the information they need. This is especially necessary with changes in the nursing staff—a new shift. Some go off duty and others come on, and he tells the new attendants of the progress his wife has made.

There is another, more subtle influence with the husband assisting his wife through childbirth. Sometimes mates feel a sense of rejection prenatally and postpartum because almost all of the wife's energy must be spent with preparation for the newborn. The new parents seemingly have no time for each other. Perhaps the two drift apart. But by working together toward the accomplishment of an easier and happier delivery, they will have achieved the goal jointly. The couple soon realizes it was their cooperation that did it, drawing them closer together.

We witnessed an occurrence where a tough, athletic outdoorsman declared himself uninterested in his wife's pregnancy. Strictly as a favor to her, he agreed to enter the delivery room and watch. He appeared bored. His attitude was that the whole thing was just a waste of his time. As soon as the obstetrician assisted the mother in the birth and was through sewing up the episiotomy, he took the baby and put it in the he-man's arms. "Here, you hold it!" the doctor said. The husband was reluctant but what could he do? He wasn't about to drop the baby on the floor. So he looked at his new daughter closely, smiled at her, talked to her, chuckled and cooed, and a bonding began right there on the spot. It made a deep impression on this man and how he was going to deal with his child from then on. That is a secondary advantage of the Bradley husband-coaching techniques. They tend to bond the father psychologically to his child.

What Makes the Bradley Method Different

In the course, Bradley instructors teach varied positions for labor. They teach how to cope with a contraction while standing or sitting on the toilet or walking from the house to the car or the car to the hospital door. They teach how to relax the body, starting from the head and working down so that all muscle groups release their tension in turn.

Diaphragmatic breathing is taught. This is natural breathing. The American Academy of Husband-Coached Childbirth believes that one cannot achieve total relaxation of every muscle using any kind of altered breathing. This idea is directly contrary to the teachings of the Dick-Read and Lamaze methods.

The Bradley method teaches that any altered breathing technique uses muscles in the thoracic cavity which forces a woman to raise her rib cage for chest breathing. "Chest breathing creates panic, tension, pain, and more chest breathing," the instructors say. This wastes energy and oxygen that could be better utilized in the uterus. In contrast, natural diaphragmatic breathing sets its own level for oxygen exchange. This will allow total relaxation of every muscle.

The Bradley proponents say, "Sleep imitation or relaxation is the key to labor. Just breathe normally. . . . 'Breathing' is an obstetrical intervention just as surely as is Demerol. People who use breathing techniques are no longer low-risk." Obviously, this line of thinking is totally different from the approaches of Dick-Read, Lamaze, Bing, and all the rest.

You learn pushing techniques such as the following: Put the head back, take two breaths, hold the second, tuck in your chin, bring up your legs, and bear down. This position eliminates the need for stirrups, since you are able to take hold of your own legs, pull them apart, hold your breath, and push. These pushing techniques are also different from other childbirth methods.

Sterile drapes are done away with as well. Bradley people believe that the baby is fairly immune to anything the mother might have. Sterile drapes are considered nothing more than bulky interference to the woman drawing back her own legs and seeing the birth of the baby from out of her own body.

You may be taught to exhale when you push. This is a technique suggested by Elizabeth Noble, RPT, author of *Essential Exercises for the Childbearing Year*, and not yet official doctrine of the American Academy of Husband-Coached Childbirth. Margaret Higle, who instructs in the Bradley technique, explained, "When you exhale with a push rather than breathhold with a push, it is much easier on the baby and on the woman. Holding the breath and then gasping for air actually draws the infant back into the birth canal. You push it out and suck it back in. Exhaling and pushing simultaneously permits movement outward only. And exhalation while pushing is more comfortable and less apt to cause you hemorrhoids."

The Bradley people teach you to practice exhaling and bearing down while having a bowel movement. "Sure enough, exhaling with a bowel movement push is much more comfortable. Try it! One does not exhaust oneself that way," said Ms. Higle. The Childbirth Education Association of Metropolitan New York does endorse exhaling and pushing simultaneously for birth of the baby.

Also in the course, you learn that labor induction is not recommended at all except for absolute medical emergency—certainly not for the convenience of the doctor—not even for the woman. An induced labor is not a natural birth, warns Ms. Higle. "Probably if you are induced or labor is augmented artificially, you won't be able to take the length and strength of the contractions without some sort of additional medication," she says.

Many hospitals have a policy of allowing labor with ruptured membranes to go no more than twenty-four hours. The main fear is of infection. This is not strictly accepted by the academy. Margaret Higle told the story of one of her students, a poorly educated eighteen-year-old easily overwhelmed by the hospital staff. The young woman and her husband, who was twenty, were innocently accepting any procedure. The young woman, who was a clinic patient, started leaking from the bag of waters, went to the twenty-four-hour limit, and was being prepared for a cesarean section. The husband, feeling uneasy about such drastic measures, telephoned for advice from Ms. Higle. She advised them to give it another hour or more before undergoing the operation. They made that request of the doctor. Then they were granted another hour. Sure enough, at the twenty-seventh hour the woman's bag of waters broke abruptly and the baby was born spontaneously in a few minutes.

At least 90 percent of the couples who go through the Bradley training are said to have a nonmedicated birth. The academy recommends that you avoid analgesia and anesthesia because it infiltrates the baby and may depress its sucking reflex, reduce cuddliness, lessen the startle reflex, affect neurological responses, and cause other harmful effects.[2] With a lumbar epidural or caudal epidural anesthetic administered, the mother cannot push on her own. Anesthesia increases the incidence of forceps delivery. A woman will not get the sensations of the birth experience which the American Academy of Husband-Coached Childbirth believes every mother should experience.

Dr. Bradley made a statement to his colleagues about the dignity of unmedicated mothers who are awake, alert, and aware. He said: "They consider the birth of their children to be a private, personal and intimate moment, to be shared with their husbands. They wisely accept hospitals as the place to bear their young, realizing that the rare complication can be handled promptly and properly, but they also recognize how much more adroitly any complication can be managed with a calm, cooperative, and grateful patient."[3]

As with other birthing methods, the proponents who put it to use, the mothers and fathers, have made modifications. In this case the academy members disagree with Dr. Bradley. They say that alternate places for birth can also be safe, such as childbirth centers and good home birth programs.

NOTES FOR CHAPTER TEN

1. Robert A. Bradley, "Father's Place During Childbirth," *Medical Opinion & Review,* December 1966.

2. Howard Fox, "Effects of Maternal Analgesia on Neonatal Morbidity." Division of Neonatal Medicine, Department of Pediatrics, University of Kansas Medical Center.

3. Bradley, "Father's Place."

11
Prenatal Yoga

*During my pregnancy my husband and I created
the "fruit method" to describe my changing
shape to friends and relatives who lived far away.
For example, at about four months I was at the
"orange" stage; at six, the "cantaloupe"; and at
nine, the "watermelon." One evening while we
were grocery shopping, my husband peeled a
RIPE sticker off an avocado and playfully placed
it on my abdomen. I must have been just that,
because four hours later I went into labor!*
—KATHY KATZ, Expecting magazine

Labor Requires Willful Relaxation

Going into labor is an ideal time to have the ability to relax at will
for relieving tension in body and mind. That willfully relaxed state is
quickly accomplished through the study of *yoga*, a discipline that goes
back to about 300 B.C. In India and other places today, yoga is practiced for purposes of centering—finding the truth within and the
meaning of life.

Originating from the Indian word *yug* meaning "bond," yoga uses
meditation, breathing techniques, and a series of physical exercises to
bond oneself to the purpose of being. In labor and delivery, the
application of yogic principles is known to release a reservoir of energy the new mother never before realized she owned. In fact, yoga
forms the basis of most of the methods of modern prepared childbirth.
The Maternity Center Association recommends it as preparation for
childbearing, as do many Lamaze and Bradley instructors.

Besides the release of nervous and muscular tension, the yoga discipline offers improved breathing and circulation; better sleep and increased vitality; an increased ability to concentrate and to cope with adverse conditions; a more balanced state of mind, at the same time feeling calmer and more alive; more erect posture; greater poise and efficient, graceful, and effortless movements. Prenatal yoga is superb preparation for giving birth.

The Seven Kinds of Yoga

There are many forms of yoga practiced, varying with the concepts of individual teachers, but seven kinds are relatively well-known and recognized internationally. Indian purists accept five of them as basic, while two others are intimately connected with the couple relationship and childbirth.

The yoga taught most frequently in the West is *hatha yoga*. It relaxes the musculature, comforts the mind, and makes one aware of his or her physical self.

Bhakta yoga teaches universal love, especially love of God. It holds that love should be given for love's sake—to each person with no fear or selfish motives and no trade-off that says, "I will love you if you will love me."

Knowledge, reason, and logic are the tools of *jnana yoga*, where the goal is to find the hub of the wheel of life from which its spokes lead us in many directions.

Karma yoga is mastery of one's self to rise above the mundane of daily living. It is a kind of action yoga that starts within and travels outward.

The highest form of the five basic yogas is *raja yoga*, that allows its disciple to master energy and achieve serenity. Its ultimate goal is the return to one's origin, the moment of resynthesis.

Tantra yoga is the transformation of sexual activity into a sacrament. By its means, ordinary mortals partake of the divine, and their sexual lives become cosmic in scope and intensity. Tantra is the yoga of sexual ecstasy—truly connected to couple intimacy.

The seventh form of yoga might seem outrageous to purists, since it tends to bastardize the high-level principles of centering that yoga teaches in general. *Eutonie yoga* is not Indian in origin at all. It was developed by Mrs. Gerda Alexander of Copenhagen, Denmark, and is the most specific for prenatal preparation. It has been used extensively in Europe as a birthing method. Alfred Bartussek, M.D., an Austrian specialist in internal medicine, says of Eutonie, "Its consequences transcend the curative effects of other systems and have an important

value for all demands made upon the human being and his (her) total
level of performance."

Prenatal Eutonie Yoga

One American graduate teacher of the eutonie method, suggests it
presents "a challenge to those who believe they are not tense and an
invitation to those who know they are." Eutonie markedly relieves tension. The technique is based on a series of exercises, which are seemingly physical. However, essentially they are different from other
ordinary exercises in that they avoid any muscular effort or strain.
Although the exercises appear physical, the effort is mental, and the
effect is both physical and emotional. Performing eutonie with certain
changes designed for pregnancy, you become aware of your body. You
enhance muscle tone and soon can better coordinate muscular exer-
tion with functional movement.

Eutonie yoga is a modification of traditional hatha yoga to make it
more beneficial for the pregnant person. Preparation includes your
"doing" a childbirth every day. The baby forming within you is
thought of as a continual pulsing manifestation of here-and-now
rhythms. The concept is that the baby looks like Buddha, an attachment within your body by means of the placenta. And later it may be
a suckling attachment to your breast—taking in nourishment and
pleasure begun with conception.

A healthy pregnancy using prenatal eutonie is accomplished in part
by believing that having a baby is having hope. The concept is that
you are recycling protoplasm. Also, it is knowing that your body, your
mind, and your spirit are perpetuating.

In practicing prenatal yoga you are engaging in spiritual preparation for the most telling event of life. That is true yoga teaching.
Practically speaking, in our opinion, it should be accompanied by
attendance at preparatory childbirth classes for physiological preparation as well.

The Philosophy of Prenatal Yoga

A philosophy for prenatal yoga says that if all men could help their
children into this world and see them emerge from their women, there
would be no more wars.

Another bit of philosophy says babies born naturally, undrugged,
and in tune to their own rhythms from whole women would provide
no stimulus for violence at all. Additionally, children of this new age

might give up our competitive, struggling, violent way of life because there would be no base in birth—no connection—to unfelt pain from which to "act out" and hurt others.

Yoga is a practice that allows you delight in being alive right now. It is a manifestation of *prana*, the primal life-force. Tension flows out of the faucet in your naval.

The discipline asks that you listen to your breathing, the *ajapna mantram*, for it is a vital nutrient nourishing the fetus and allowing your uterus to grow.

One prenatal yoga practitioner described how and where she partakes in the discipline's philosophy: "At the ocean today, belly bare—I sat in the pushing posture of childbirth and drew up my skirt—legs open, facing the sun and the clear sea. I felt the waters within my womb flow out to the expansiveness of the ocean—and the ocean flow into my vagina to merge with the amniotic fluids in which my baby now lives. This oneness was ecstatic. My womb felt akin to the ocean —we both are containers, bringing forth beginnings and new life; I felt the power of my uterus and the sea, delighted in our rhythms, our changing forms and our infiniteness."

Varieties of Yoga Exercises

Yoga exercises include standing tall to feel your tailbone drawn to the center of the earth to the origin of the *kundalini* power within. The kundalini is said to be a mysterious psychic energy often referred to as "serpent power" because in its quiescent form, it lies coiled around the base of the spinal column. Tantric yoga describes it as "luminous as lightning, shining in the hollow of this lotus like a chain of brilliant lights."

Tantric yoga also says that the kind of breath flow of the parents during intercourse will determine the sex of the child, if conception occurs. Thus, if the man's breath is through the *pingala* or right nostril, and the woman's through the *ida* or left nostril, the resulting child will be a male. The converse being true, the child will be a girl. If both parents are in the same nostril breath, Tantric doctrine says the child will be predisposed to homosexuality.

Hatha yoga asks you to feel the top of your head drawn upward and expanding in all directions. Rock back and forth to locate the center of life. See your legs as roots of a mighty tree firmly grounded. Exercise your neck in a revolution to draw a circle of white light with the beam you imagine coming out of the top of your head. Use balance and symmetry in your exercising. Seven neck rolls to the left require seven neck rolls to the right.

All of the yoga disciplines require that you do squats. Bend your knees to avoid stress on the backs of your legs. Feel the life flow in this bioenergetic posture. Feel warmth with the flow of energy. Do everything in slow motion. Feel peace and well-being inside you as you go through the movements.

There are many exercise forms in yoga, including standing *kundalini shakti* that we have just described—the inner thigh stretch, lunges, the thunderbolt posture, the pendulum-diaphragm stretch, the mountain pose, pelvic rocks, the dog tail wag, the python, the centaur, pelvis leg lifts, the hiss breath, and the camel. Breathing exercises consist of the puff breath, the moon-sun breath, progressive relaxation, and yoga meditation. Here we will only describe the specific eutonie techniques appropriate to the prenatal period.

Prenatal Exercises of the Eutonie Method

Mrs. Joop Gomperts, a Danish-trained eutonie instructor (now retired), gave us information about the prenatal exercises with their modifications from the eutonie method. Mrs. Gomperts specified rules to be followed with prenatal eutonie: do not perform sit-up exercises, avoid facedown positions, allow no strain of the abdomen, and don't assume *forced* postures that demand forward bending or upward stretching. You can do a few of the bending or stretching exercises noted below that are unforced.

The following are some of the eutonie exercises recommended as advantageous in pregnancy and as preparation for labor and delivery:

1. Sit cross-legged on the floor in the tailor position (Figure 22).
2. Sit on heels and knees, bend together without forcing, so that your head rests on the floor (Figure 23). Watch your breathing and imagine you are breathing through the tailbone.
3. Perform a pelvic rock on the hands and knees and arch the lower back up and down (Figure 24). Do not overstretch.
4. Sit on a stool as high as your knees. Focus attention on your back and feel free and untense. Mentally order your shoulders to sink backward and down (Figure 25).
5. Sit on the floor with knees apart and soles together. Fold hands around the head and bend forward gently as far as possible without strain. Let the weight of the arms pull your body forward down (Figure 26).
6. Merely sit on the floor with legs stretched and wide apart and meditate (Figure 27).
7. Do the "dog stretch" by sitting on the heels and knees, bent to-

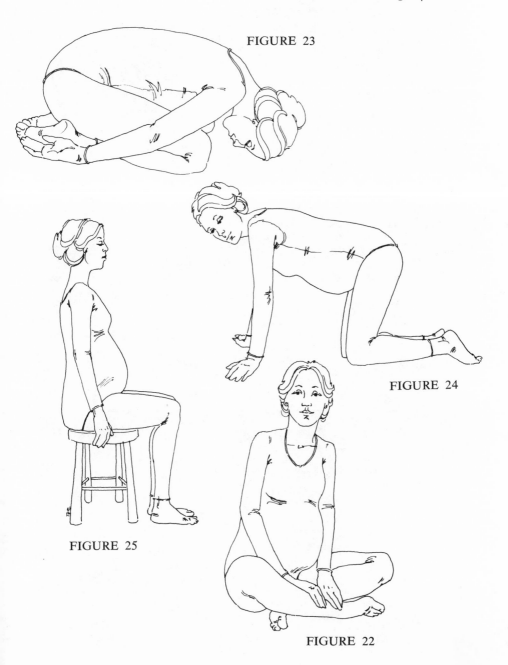

FIGURE 23

FIGURE 24

FIGURE 25

FIGURE 22

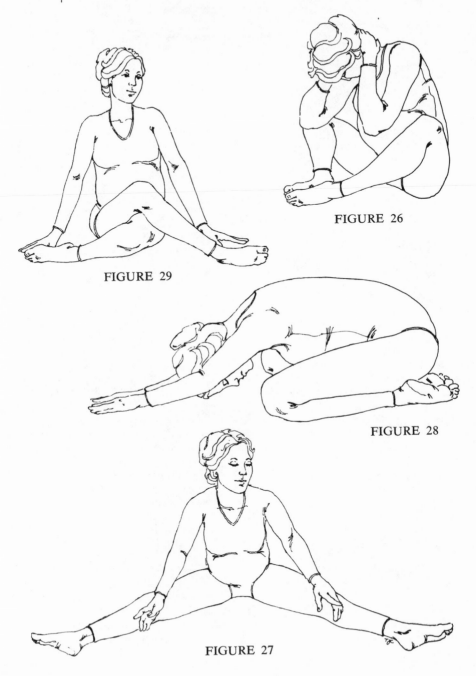

FIGURE 29

FIGURE 26

FIGURE 28

FIGURE 27

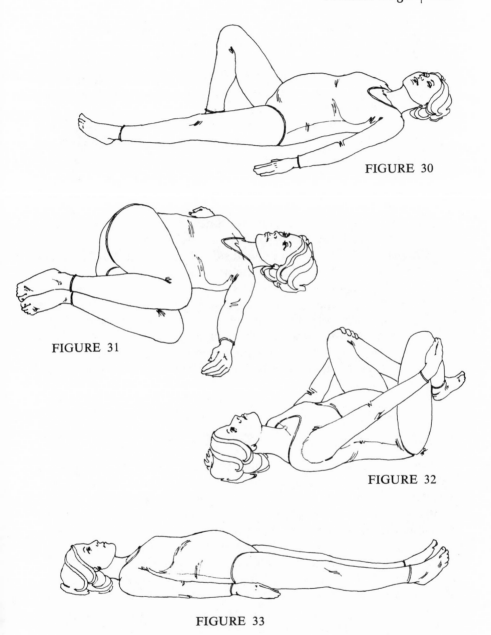

FIGURE 30

FIGURE 31

FIGURE 32

FIGURE 33

gether so that the head rests on the floor and the arms are out-stretched in front. Lift the buttocks and let the arms slide forward, drawing the body with them (Figure 28).

8. Do the "scissors" by sitting with the right knee bent up as in the tailor position. Place the left leg under the right so that one knee is above the other (Figure 29).

9. Outstretched on the back, bend the right knee outward and backward so that lower leg is as close to the thigh as possible. Keep back flat (Figure 30).

10. Lie on the back with knees bent to the side and soles of the feet together. Let knees sink by their own weight toward the floor (Figure 31).

11. While still on the back, bend the knees toward the breast. Hold each knee with the hands from the inside and let them fall apart. Concentrate on releasing the inside thigh muscles so that the knees sink toward the floor (Figure 32).

12. Lie on the floor with a tennis ball under one side of the back between the spine and the shoulder blade. Use the ball as a focus for your concentration, yield to the pressure, and picture your back sinking down on the ball. After a few minutes, when you do not feel the ball anymore, remove it. You can also use two balls at the same time, one under each side of the spine (Figure 33).

Lorraine Kweskin's Experience with Yoga for Childbirth

"When I first started with eutonie yoga I was not yet pregnant. In fact, I did not go through any formal yoga training for pregnancy. The eutonie, however, had me in fairly good physical shape, and my entire pregnancy experience was pleasant," said Mrs. Lorraine Kweskin, the mother of three children.

"That yoga training definitely made it easier for me to have my first child, even though I had attended no preparatory classes in childbirth. I had gone into labor concentrating on the deep breathing techniques and relaxation methods I had learned in eutonie. I never knew what was going to happen next—not the stages of labor or anything—but yoga principles kept me from losing control. I was not afraid of what was happening, and I did float with it," Mrs. Kweskin said.

"I employed my prenatal yoga for day-to-day activities. I could pick up objects without straining because eutonie training had taught me how. All of the principles of relaxation came into play—without fatigue and without imposing unnecessary pressures on me. In addition, yoga principles of relaxation have been useful for me throughout life," she said. "I would have labor and delivery this way again, except I would take prepared childbirth instruction, as was the case with my third pregnancy. To know what is going to happen is very important; it's such a secure, nice feeling.

"Finally, the closest anyone might come to having 'natural' childbirth as women did many years ago, or do today in Third World countries, is to give birth merely employing the principles of 'yoga childbirth,' " Mrs. Kweskin concluded.

Pre- and Postnatal Yoga Information Sources

Two books will make available many more yoga exercises and breathing techniques than are annotated here. Judi Thompson has written *Healthy Pregnancy the Yoga Way*[1] and Jeannine O'Brien Medvin is the author of *Prenatal Yoga*.[2] Neither book, however, describes the method of eutonie yoga. For that information you will have to get instructions directly from a eutonie teacher in your area.

An organization devoted to herbal, spiritual, and yogic techniques for childbirth gives counseling for a holistic prenatal approach in a clinic called the "Birth and Death Center." For information about prenatal yoga write to Jeannine O'Brien Medvin, the executive director of The Center for Family Growth, 555 Highland Avenue, Cototi, California 94928.

NOTES FOR CHAPTER ELEVEN

1. Judi Thompson, *Healthy Pregnancy the Yoga Way* (New York: Doubleday and Co., 1977).
2. Jeannine O'Brien Medvin, *Prenatal Yoga and Natural Birth* (Albion, Calif.: Freestone Publishing Co., 1975).

๙ 12

Acupuncture
for Pregnancy

The Variable Methods of Medicine

There are some unusual phenomena in medicine. The most curious perhaps is acupuncture, including its ability to take away pain through the insertion of a needle into a part of the body seemingly unrelated to the area that hurts. One might wonder if this is some new medical marvel when, in truth, the practice goes back beyond the third millennium B.C. Chinese doctors in 1971 created quite a stir among visitors from the West by reopening mainland China and letting them see treatments and surgery performed with the aid of acupuncture and no other means of eliminating pain.

How and why does the phenomenon take place? It seems to occur by the simple alternation of electrical charges in the nerves affected by the acupuncture needles. Some form of energy present in the body, possibly electricity, is indicated by measuring devices to detect its frequencies. The Chinese call it *Ch'i* (pronounced *Chee* and also spelled Tch'i) and consider it the life-force. Western scientists already have stimulated the larger nerves of the body to block pain impulses emitted from their tributaries by altering *Ch'i* with engineering technology.

The Chinese say that this life-force energy is governed by two antagonistic and complementary principles, yin and yang. *Yin* is feminine and *yang* is masculine. They are present in each of us, with one slightly predominating, according to your sex.

There is a single, absolute law in Chinese medicine: The universe is the oscillation of the two activities, yin and yang, and its vicissitudes. When they are out of harmony—more of one present than the other —the body imbalance manifests itself in illness or *dis-ease*. Thus, some yin is present in yang, and vice versa. One is dependent on and equal to the other, and each flows into the other, similar to day flowing into night, and night into day. Block this flow and you will alter the life-force.

How Does It Work?

Where do the needles come in? You have good reason to ask! The Chinese discovered that energy flows all through the human body along definite lines called *meridians*. The study of these meridians over hundreds of years determined that the life-force energy flow on the inner side of the limbs is yin and the flow on the outer side is yang.

Twelve meridians course through the body, plus two median lines. One median line for *conception* is located on the front of the head and trunk, and the other which governs *flow* is located on the back. The median line we are most concerned with—the conception vessel—acts on the respiratory, digestive, and urogenital systems. It is totally responsible for reproduction and all the acts in the drama of childbirth.

Vital energy is most apparent in this reproductive median line, known as the *triple warming meridian*, between 9:00 P.M. and 11:00 P.M. Therefore, if you are anxious to conceive, the acupunturists recommend this two-hour period as the best time to have sexual intercourse.

According to Yiwen Y. Tang, M.D., a Harvard-trained physician and former president of the Pacific Coast Chapter of the American Acupuncture Society, "a single needle can free the body from ten thousand maladies." The trick is to know where to put the needle.

Another part of the trick is to know the correct time. As we indicated, certain organs are at their nadir of energy at different times of the day. The way the needle is manipulated affects the organ, too.

Nobody knows precisely how many acupuncture points there are in the entire body. Varying numbers—500, 785, 824 points—have been located by a bevy of acupuncturists. However, the points for pregnancy and relief for its symptoms of discomfort have been decided upon. Dr. Tang admits that we in the West don't know why they relieve labor pain, but they do.

There are dangers, of course. In the hands of an unskilled practitioner, the area he is attempting to sedate might accidentally be stimulated. It is possible to cause an abortion. "I'm terrified that many doctors with limited or practically no knowledge will attempt to use acupuncture for a therapeutic effect, and a lot of damage will be done," warned Dr. Kenneth Riland, who visited China with President Nixon in February 1972.

Acupuncture Really Does Work for Childbirth

President Nixon's personal physician, Major General Walter R. Tkach, U.S. Air Force, was enormously impressed by what he saw during that 1972 trip. "They have something very superior to our method of anesthesia," Dr. Tkach concluded. "It's something we had better learn about and make use of clinically as a possible whole new kind of anesthetic."

Ear surgeon Samuel Rosen, M.D., emeritus professor at New York's Mount Sinai School of Medicine, wrote in *The New York Times* on November 1, 1971, "I have seen the past and it works!" He gave a glowing report of the use of acupuncture for medical and surgical procedures. He had witnessed them earlier in China, in the company of the late, famed cardiologist Paul Dudley White, M.D., and two other doctors. One of them was Victor Sidel, M.D., a specialist in social and community medicine. In a lecture to the American Medical Writers Association, Dr. Sidel described case histories where acupuncture was used as the anesthetic of choice for labor and delivery. The procedures were totally drugless and harmless, he said.

More recent American medical visitors to China have come away amazed at what they saw. Ralph Gause, M.D., a former chief of obstetrics and gynecology, Roosevelt Hospital, New York, and currently a consultant to Planned Parenthood in Vermont and to the State Board of Health in Mississippi, spent seventeen days observing family planning and women's health care in China. He returned from his trip in the fall, 1977 with great respect for Chinese achievements in general and a feeling that the United States can improve. One day Dr. Gause observed a typical sterilization procedure, a hysterectomy, and a cesarean section taking only fourteen minutes (see Chapter 22). All were performed under acupuncture.

"Acupuncture is the anesthesia of choice, and it seems to work beautifully. I do not know if any preoperative medication was given the hysterectomy patient because I did not see the beginning of the procedure, but acupuncture was all that was necessary for the other two," Dr. Gause said.

One of the research priorities in China is to discover why acupuncture works so well, he noted.[1]

Dr. Tang assured us that in 1949 he was able to give comfort "to quite a few patients using acupuncture. Needling helped them to relax, kept them calm, and conditioned them to accept labor pain, if it was present. However, with the current methods of natural childbirth which work so well without drugs or needles, I do not see much future in the continued use of acupuncture for labor and delivery in the United States. It seems unnecessary. I think other things are more important for our women—education about childbirth, excellent nutrition before and during pregnancy, and good physical fitness. My belief is that one's health does not start from the day you are born, it starts from the moment you are conceived."

The Techniques of Acupuncture

"The needles are of varying lengths," said Ellen F. Leong, M.D., a member of the New York Society of Acupuncture for Physicians and Dentists. "Soft tissue density determines how long the needle used will be. For needling an acupuncture point in the ear, perhaps the one-half-inch length will be required, but in very fleshy areas a four-inch needle might be required. The needles are of different gauges from number 34 or number 32 for the shorter ones (the higher the number, the finer the gauge) to as thick as number 28 for the longest one. The gold needle is for tonifying the tissues, the silver needle is for sedating, although stainless steel is the general all-purpose metal employed. But in the final analysis, the doctor's judgment is what determines the places and purposes of needle insertion. Local and distant points are pierced, since each has its own property," the acupuncturist said.

"In pregnancy," Dr. Leong continued, "there are several points employed to relieve uterine pain, to help the uterus contract, and to speed labor. I give acupuncture for obstetrics to my own patients but not for another physician's patients. Individual doctors should take acupuncture courses in order to make obstetrical application. The acupuncture procedure is begun for a pregnant woman at the beginning of the thirty-seventh week so as to condition her body in advance. Doing this about three weeks prior to labor and delivery tends to shorten the actual labor period."

The reproductive organs are composed of sensitive nerves. For the ovaries, fallopian tubes, and uterus, the local contacts are located across the lower abdomen near each pubic bone where they come together. There are more distant points that affect labor—the foot, the hand, each side of the knee, and the low back, for instance. Also difficulties with postpartum pain and dysmenorrhea (difficult and painful menstruation) are benefited by acupuncture treatment.

Aquapuncture: A Variation for Women in Labor

Because an acupuncturist fears that a woman in labor will thrash about excessively and break the inserted needles, he or she may give the patient aquapuncture. *Aquapuncture* is the practice of injecting soluble vitamins of the B complex into the appropriate sites for affecting the life-force flowing through the reproductive meridian. Vitamin B_1, vitamin B_6, vitamin B_{12}, or just saline (salt solution) is injected into the acupuncture points to stimulate them. Aquapuncture avoids the danger of needle breakage in the body during very severe labor contractions by a quick injection of the liquid vitamin. It remains at the injection site for a short time as if the needle has been left in place. Aquapuncture is therefore a substitute for acupuncture for pregnancy.

Incidentally, Chinese acupuncture sites are not numbered. Instead they are given names such as "Heavenly Ravine," "Cloud Gate," "Welcome Sweet Small," "Fountainhead," and others. The health of the fetus and pregnant person can be ensured by the points' special functions on muscles—some tonify, some sedate, and others harmonize forces within the body. American acupuncture experts have made judgments about the old Asian science and modernized it. That is where injecting vitamins comes in.

Acupressure—a Further Step

Acupressure is another form that is used. What is acupressure? Any good book on physics will tell you that energy cannot be destroyed but it can travel; it cannot be seen, since it is invisible, but it can leave the body. As it leaves the body, the person gets weaker and weaker. The heart is the generator for the electricity in the body. If you have ever talked with anyone who has had a heart attack, he will tell you that his energy just seemed to drain away.

Acupressure restores that energy and is especially useful near the end of labor. A woman can actually become revitalized by correct acupressure application. It is slower than acupuncture and requires much repetition of contact with the tip of the index and third fingers, or, for more strength, the index finger reinforced by the third finger placed on top. Pressure is applied to the energy centers affecting the reproductive organs. The pressure should be firm but not hard enough to be acutely painful. A doctor or midwife employing acupuncture will know the acupressure points and be able to educate the new mother's coach-assistant for longer and frequent applications.

Acupuncture and its sister science acupressure are proven systems used for centuries by the Asians to create a smooth flow of vibratory energy throughout the body. We have explained that the acupuncturist contacts various points on the pathways which relate to the organs, glands, and cells, usually with the use of steel needles inserted at certain spots. This is done for one more reason: the body not only is electrical in nature, but it has its positive and negative poles. The heart represents the negative; the brain on the right side represents the positive. The old Chinese teachings say that there should be balance between the heart and the brain.

Dr. Leong Describes an Acupuncture Delivery

Dr. Leong told us of several childbirths for which she employed acupuncture. One Asian woman pregnant with her first baby came for prenatal care regularly and took the usual acupuncture treatment after her thirty-sixth week. "At each visit she was quiet and uncommunicative, but in labor she became fearful, nervous, and hysterical. When I arrived on the scene the hospital admitting staff prepared me for my patient's crying and yelling. I spoke to her and explained the whole technique of acupuncture—how it works and why and that the acupuncture would prevent any additional discomfort. This educational talk tended to calm her. She needed only to understand. Then I proceeded with my needling technique," Dr. Leong said. "With each puncture I verbally reinforced the idea of how it takes away pain.

"When my patient was four centimeters dilated I asked if her contractions were painful, and she said, 'I'm fine.' The woman had received no sedation at all. I told her how to breathe, since she had been exposed to no previous instruction for prepared childbirth," Dr. Leong told us. "Her labor went quickly and really good contractions came upon her.

"Again I asked how she was feeling. I offered sedation for pain, but it was refused. My questioning continued from time to time, and all the while she said that the contractions gave her no discomfort at all. She said, 'It gets hard in my tummy, that's all!'

"I was happy that with each passing minute the woman was coming closer to giving birth, but I wasn't sure about her freedom from pain. It was, after all, her first pregnancy. I kept offering sedation by injection and she kept turning me down. At six centimeters dilation, upon being offered injection sedation again, she replied, 'No, I hate injections, the acupuncture is working fine.'

"Pretty soon she was fully dilated and pushing. We wheeled her into the delivery room where I thought she might need some gas to put her to sleep. I told the anesthetist to place the mask over her face. 'What's that?' my patient yelled. I explained it was gas to eliminate discomfort. She repeated that there was absolutely no pain and she wanted no gas. I said O.K.!

"Then I informed her that I was going to give her a local anesthetic down below. 'For what?' she asked. I explained, 'I'm going to cut you for the episiotomy.' She answered, 'You go ahead and cut, and if it hurts I'll let you know.' She watched in the overhead mirror and never made a move. The baby was delivered with some difficulty. Again I said that I had to put a local anesthetic in there in order to sew up the episiotomy. 'Don't inject me,' she said. 'Just sew up the cut. I'll tell you if it hurts!' It did not.

"The next morning while my patient walked up and down the hall, she asked me why it bothered her a bit down below. I think the acupuncture may have worn off," concluded Dr. Leong. "I explained the situation and my patient accepted it without another thought given to it."

NOTES FOR CHAPTER TWELVE

1. Fran Pollner, "China's Success Hard to Duplicate Here, Ob. Gyn. Says," *Obstetrics and Gynecology News,* October 15, 1977.

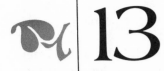 **13**

An Obstetrical Trance Through Hypnotherapy

I decided to have a baby and it turned out to be the best resolution of my life. Now I'm totally entranced by my child's delight in the world. Seeing things through her eyes has rekindled my love of living.

—BETSEY JOHNSON, *a maternity and children's fashion designer,* Boston Globe

Acupuncture May Be Some Form of Medical Hypnotism

From the previous chapter, perhaps you took note that the doctor verbally conditions his or her patient prior to acupuncture application. It has been observed that Chinese acupuncturists spend a lot of time in "philosophical discussions" with obstetrical and surgical patients, "preparing" them for what is to come. In China, patients are seen clutching their *Little Red Book* of Chairman Mao's thoughts during operations. This tends to qualify acupuncture as some form of medical hypnosis or autosuggestion.

During hypnosis there is a decline in heartbeat, respiration rate, oxygen consumption, carbon dioxide elimination, blood lactate, and blood pressure, accompanied by a rise in electrical skin resistance and intensity of alpha brain waves. Some of this alteration in human system functioning is advantageous for the easing of the birth process. Alpha-brain-wave intensity is known to enter into the success of inward turning characteristic of the Grantly Dick-Read childbirth approach. And Dr. Dick-Read has been hard pressed by his detractors to prove that his method was not actually another form of obstetrical trance through hypnotherapy, no different from what people had been exposed to as entertainment in the theater.

The average lay person's concept of hypnosis probably stems from having seen a stage hypnotist inducing people to make fools of themselves ("Whenever I scratch my head, you will bark like a dog"). Medical hypnotism is quite another matter. "Hypnotism acts as a splint on the mind," says Abraham Weinberg, M.D., who uses the trance state to assist in obstetrics.

A report by the American Medical Association Council on Mental Health published in the *Journal of the American Medical Association* (September 13, 1958) advises that hypnotism should be used "on a highly selective basis" and should never become the single technique employed for therapy or childbirth, lest other "conditions" arise.

The deep, sleeplike trance is used only occasionally as an anesthetic in obstetrics. Why is it not routine? Because not everyone can be hypnotized. It is estimated that a deep trance can be induced in only 5 percent of the population, a medium trance in about 35 percent, and a light trance in most of the balance of people. Some authorities argue that many individuals walk around in a partial hypnotic state all the time, but that has never been verified. If you are one of those who are able to achieve the deepest sleeplike stage, you may be able to engage in obstetrical hypnotherapy. It has its benefits.

The Benefits of Hypnotherapy for Childbirth

In Denver, obstetricians have been using hypnotherapy to speed the healing of episiotomies and other surgical wounds.

Herbert Benson, M.D., and Robert Keith Wallace, Ph.D., published a report that said: ". . . in a hypnotized subject, the brain-wave activity takes the form characteristic of the mental state that has been suggested to the subject." Thus, if you are in labor while settled into a deep trance, your obstetrician can make the experience quite comfortable simply by painting a picture in your mind that is most pleasant. Beforehand, you and the doctor may have decided what that scene and situation might be, and you can be made to relive it throughout the birthing experience. As we shall explain later, you are able to switch your pleasant scene on and off at will, in accordance with the frequency and severity of labor contractions.

An anesthetic effect is readily achieved, without drugs, by the use of hypnotic suggestion alone. It is obtained through control of a person's pain sense. She will refuse to recognize any nerve impulses which ordinarily would lead to discomfort. In that way, the nerve messages from labor contractions which would normally register as a sensation of pain are denied by the subject—she refuses to recognize them. Any labor pain is inconsistent with the already accepted generalization of anesthesia.

Controlling any discomfort can be continued as long as the hypnotizing doctor (or other assisting person) deems it necessary. The suggestion of comfort will be accepted by the subject, and will have a generalization effect.

Posthypnotic suggestions can be given to make a woman oblivious to any discomforts felt during the pregnancy, delivery or postdelivery. For example, episiotomy or some other irritation will be ignored simply because the irritation is not felt.

Postpartum "blues" can be prevented through suggestion while the mother is in the sleeping state.

Indeed, all kinds of advantageous posthypnotic suggestions may be offered to overcome undesirable traits such as:

Overanxiety	Functional hypertension
Fears and phobias	Nervous headaches
Hypochondria	Personality defects
Compulsions	Nervous habits
Obsessions	Hallucinations
Depressions	Delusions
Neurotic disturbances and other disturbances	

There are no dangers, discomforts, or disadvantages to being hypnotized for childbearing. However, it does require much more time than some women or obstetricians are willing to invest. Twenty minutes to an hour can be used up during the first office visit to induce an initial trance. This first trance will probably be performed the sixth month of pregnancy and will be followed up with reinduction on each succeeding prenatal visit. Hypnotic induction gets easier the more you go under.

Requirements for Obstetrical Hypnosis

In addition to having a coaching assistant or physician who knows how to induce a trance, what else is required for the use of hypnosis as your form of obstetrical procedure? Usually nothing more than the willingness to undergo the hypnotic induction. Your personal motivation and interpersonal communication with your physician are the two primary factors for successful application of this method for child-birth.

The physician who employs obstetrical hypnosis will probably give you a susceptibility test in the sixth prenatal month. The technique of medical relaxation with susceptibility testing is common in the health professions. Dentists apply it frequently for highly apprehensive people who are afraid of being subjected to pain, no matter how minor the dental procedure.

A susceptibility test involves having you listen to the relaxing words of the doctor. While sitting comfortably with both feet on the floor, you may be asked to close your eyes, extend your arms in front of you with palms down, and imagine that your hands are holding heavy weights. The susceptibility test will have proved successful if you were, indeed, able to feel the heaviness of the weights dragging down on your arms. At the same time, you may have discovered that exercising your imagination in that way was rather relaxing. This comfortable sensation means that you have experienced the lightest stage of hypnosis—medical relaxation.

Most often it is a good feeling and you may immediately be inclined to proceed with hypnotic suggestions as the childbirth method of choice. Your doctor will take it from there, if he or she is trained in the techniques of autohypnosis for delivering babies.

In 1961, the AMA Council on Mental Health recommended that 144 hours of training be given to physicians interested in medical hypnosis over a nine- to twelve-month period at the undergraduate and postgraduate levels. For information about a physician who may use hypnosis for obstetrics contact either of two professional organizations: The American Society for Clinical Hypnosis and the International Society of Clinical and Experimental Hypnosis. Both have established sections in many countries throughout the world. There may be one near you. Write to them care of the American Medical Association, 535 North Dearborn Street, Chicago, Illinois 06010. Telephone (312) 751-6000. Cable address: "Medic" Chicago.

A Physician Speaks on Delivery with Hypnosis

"My technique for rendering obstetrical service under hypnosis was to teach the patient to put herself under at will. During the period of pregnancy, I preconditioned my patient. First I preconditioned her for hypnotic induction by external control—me—and then I preconditioned her to go into self-hypnosis—internal control—and institute her own relaxation technique.

"The woman's personal relaxation technique allows just the uterus to contract and not her entire muscular structure. In pelvic relaxation, the pelvic bones move apart, the cervix dilates, and the baby comes down through the birth canal with a lot less trouble," said Harold W. Harper, M.D. in an interview. Dr. Harper is a specialist in holistic medicine and orthomolecular nutrition who has delivered hundreds of babies but doesn't offer obstetrical service anymore. He is an active member of the American College of Medical Hypnotists, where he took training in autohypnosis and self-suggestion for obstetrics.

"I delivered a woman under hypnosis at the same time my first wife was in labor with our fourth child," he told us. "Of course, my wife was being treated by another physician. She was in labor for twelve hours and had labor pains the whole time. Her obstetrician had to give her scopolamine to bring on twilight sleep so that she could give birth. On the other hand, I was delivering my patient of her second child, and she labored with no pain under hypnosis for only six hours. My patient received no anesthesia, no predelivery preparation, no analgesia of any kind, and she was awake and aware the whole time. I can't say the same thing for my wife. She had plenty of pain and had to be put to sleep.

"My patient used self-hypnosis," said Dr. Harper. "Anytime she felt a contraction coming on she just put herself under hypnosis—snap, like that! It was a matter of autosuggestion that I had taught her from three to five months before, during our initial consultation for hypnosis training. That training visit took about thirty minutes of office time."

Dr. Harper's method, one recommended by the American College of Medical Hypnotists, is to precondition the susceptible patient to go into anesthetic relaxation from the waist down. Pain is a concept that can be turned on, say the hypnotists, but an individual can be taught to undergo a brain switch by the use of some key phrase or suggestive word that turns off the pain. For example, Dr. Harper's obstetrical patients would tell themselves, "I am cold and numb from my waist down!" This sentence was the suggestion switch that turned off pain as the uterine contraction came on. He taught his pregnant patients the technique at the first consultation for hypnotic training, and then the women practiced on their own at home every day and demonstrated their autosuggestion ability to the physician upon visiting him for their routine prenatal checkup. His testing technique consisted of the patient numbing her limb and watching the doctor stick it with a needle. She felt no pain, and this tended to reinforce her self-confidence in her own autosuggestion ability. As a woman got better at self-hypnosis, relaxation came easier, until it could be accomplished in seconds.

"The patient I delivered when my wife was hospitalized for our fourth child gave birth to a baby whose head was hardly molded at all.

This is good because it means the baby was subjected to no trauma. There were other benefits she experienced. We used hypnosis for her episiotomy; no local anesthetic was needed. She had practiced faithfully and assisted herself in the labor and delivery.

"Thus, the mother was not the only beneficiary of the hypnotic technique," Dr. Harper pointed out. "Her baby was subjected to no drugs whatsoever. I can't say the same for my child."

The One Disadvantage of Obstetrical Hypnosis

As with any method, there is bound to be one big disadvantage of having hypnosis as your method of childbirth. The disadvantage of individualized obstetrical hypnosis is high cost! It becomes very consuming of the doctor's time if a full course of hypnosis is given each time the patient makes a prenatal visit. It would financially ruin a family with an average income, or at least make the cost of childbirth disproportionately high. Economically, therefore, it is not feasible to have the medical hypnotist administer hypnosis periodically and all through labor.

That disadvantage can be overcome by picking up on the method employed by Dr. Harper. The patient must do a daily practice session of autosuggestion at home. It is a simple, sound, and convenient procedure that fits easily into today's common practice of taking time out for twenty minutes twice a day for transcendental meditation or some other form of mind control. The autosuggestion procedure takes only five minutes a day.

Autosuggestion During Pregnancy

Autosuggestion involves the conscious process of silently repeating a phrase to yourself to achieve the desired physical or mental state. For example, Emile Coué (1857–1926) recommended a formula for autosuggestion that brought a healthy attitude to millions: "Every day, in every way, I am getting better and better."

This form of self-hypnosis accomplishes its effect in the waking state. It does not require that you go to sleep or that you become under the control of another person outside yourself. You maintain yourself as your own control. The phrase or sentence becomes the switch that helps you go into the trance state with your eyes open and mind awake to anything happening around you.

An additional way to achieve autosuggestion is to tell yourself what you want to achieve when you are just dropping off to sleep. At that time you will be talking to your subconscious as well as the conscious mind, two parts of you that will take control and rule your body when you need and want control. In that manner, you will be giving yourself posthypnotic suggestions two ways: conscious mental repetition of the key phrase that says what you want to achieve and subconscious communication with your autonomic nervous system.

At the same time that you repeat your key phrase, perform deep breathing. For some women the deep breathing alone is enough to trigger the desired numbing effect when the thought strikes their subconscious simultaneously. You will find this autosuggestion method applicable to conquering almost any exercise of the mind throughout your entire life, not only for delivering a baby.

14

The Decompression Birthing Bubble

The way we give birth to our young is that the muscular organ in which the offspring has been nurtured for nine months begins to contract. The contractions work to open the neck of the uterus and then expel the baby and the nourishing organ down the birth canal and out through the vaginal opening. This process, which pushes the baby out of its warm, wet, nearly dark, and rhythmically rocking home is as complicated a physical drama as humans are likely to be able to witness. At the same time, it is a simple miracle. We call it labor.
—REBECCA ROWE PARFITT,
The Birth Primer

Labor Can Be Eased with Decompression

Decompression during labor is another illustration of medical technology's plunge into the machine age. And while it tends to remove childbirth from an event directed by nature, labor may be eased with the use of decompression.

What is the decompression process? It is the mechanical easing of the surrounding atmospheric pressure on the external wall of the pregnant abdomen so that the wall can more easily stretch to accommodate the growing baby. Decompression also removes the weight of internal adjacent structures from the contracting uterus. The atmospheric pressure on one's abdominal area at sea level is equivalent to one thousand pounds of weight. If this weight is removed while a woman is undergoing a labor contraction, you can see that all of her contractual effort can be dedicated to expulsion of the fetus from the uterus and out through the birth canal, rather than using that effort to lift the uterine wall against pressure. The birthing process is bound to move along faster and end sooner that way.

Furthermore, with less resistance being offered to the uterus by the abdominal walls, each contraction will take place possibly with less pain. The uterus can expand or reduce without external pressure. Contractions are able to build up unrestricted and come to an end much faster. Because there were no restrictions present, some mothers have said that the pain is entirely removed. They have completely enjoyed the use of decompression technology.

Another thing, some doctors have reported that pressure reduction within the uterus brings in an extra oxygen supply to the fetus—blood circulation improves through the placenta.[1]

The Method of Decompression Delivery

Decompression against the abdominal walls is delivered by an extraabdominal decompression pump that looks like an oversized vacuum cleaner. It forms an airtight space above the protruding abdomen by means of a large, plastic Styrofoam shell or "bubble," padded at the edges with foam rubber. The shell is lightweight and pliable to conform comfortably to an individual's contours. It comes in three sizes to fit different abdominal areas. Plastic sheeting fitted snuggly around both the body of the patient and the bubble ensures the vacuum seal. A hose connects this bubble to a suction pump. When the suction pump turns on, air is withdrawn from the bubble space through a negative-pressure action, and the pregnant woman's abdominal wall is lifted. To examine the patient the nursing personnel or doctor can easily lift off the bubble with one hand. Holding the machine's microswitch in her hand, the pump turns on when the patient presses the switch just before or during a contraction. The pump takes action at once. Twenty to twenty-five pounds of negative pressure lifts your abdominal wall, allowing the uterus to contract more efficiently. You can adjust the amount of pressure by turning a dial. The decompression effect continues forty-five to sixty seconds, as long as the length of a usual contraction.

The decompression birthing bubble is just a mechanical method of contraction control, similar to those techniques of the various prepared childbirth procedures.

Nurses such as Lynne Bisceglia, R.N., and Evelyn Mish, R.N., who tend to women in hospital maternity sections, are quite enthusiastic about the advantageous effects of the decompression birthing bubble. Mrs. Mish, head nurse in the obstetrical department at Saint Joseph Hospital in Stamford, Connecticut, said, "This baby bubble is really a modification of the Grantly Dick-Read method of breathing. It encourages breath control with the abdomen in contradistinction to the Lamaze method that requires chest puffing and blowing. In my experience, this decompression bubble is excellent as a way to move along dilation of the cervix, especially for *primigravidas* [women who are pregnant for the first time]. Not only that, it keeps them occupied psychologically—something to do besides concentrating on labor pain. Our patients don't panic when using the birthing machine," she said.

"We have found it very beneficial at Saint Joseph Hospital for years. But now with almost everyone attending childbirth preparation classes, the baby bubble is coming into disuse. Using the machine for anyone in labor, including a *multipara* [a woman who has had two or more children] who never had childbirth education, will have that woman notice a remarkable difference from her prior births to this one with the bubble. Women tell me there is definite relief from contraction discomfort; labor speeds up, too. The bubble brings about better relaxation, and there is less requirement for medication," said Nurse Mish. "Sometimes just one dose of sedative medication is insufficient and a woman will require more. But if my patient is using this birthing bubble, no additional medication is necessary.

"In fact, some of the girls get so attached to using the birthing machine that they want to take it into the delivery room while it sits on their abdomens. Of course, they cannot do so. It is a fire hazard because the machine is not grounded, and it can't be used in the presence of oxygen and anesthesia.

"It made my job as head maternity nurse much easier those days when we were busy on the maternity floor. Now the number of births have diminished or leveled off and we aren't so rushed with many deliveries anymore. The birthing bubble kept the women busy then and reminded them to time their contractions. We have used the bubble for labor for at least ten years," the obstetrical nurse explained. "And when the husbands began to be allowed into the labor room, around 1969, they pushed the microswitch for their wives when asked to do so.

"The only disadvantage I found was its use for a woman with a high threshold of pain. The woman can take a lot. When that's the case, you can't tell how advanced toward delivery she is because the pressure of her contraction is almost completely relieved for her by the machine," said Evelyn Mish, R.N.

"The baby bubble is not very effective for back labor, though," put in Nurse Lynne Bisceglia. "I love the idea of the bubble because I have seen that it definitely speeds along labor, and it helps the patient stay in control. It cuts down on the amount of needed medication, too. I'm a firm believer in its use. Unfortunately for myself, I experienced posterior labor. The baby bubble doesn't do anything much for you when labor is in the back."

Origins of Decompression for Obstetrics

The discoverer of abdominal decompression was O. S. Heyns, D.Sc., a Fellow of the British Royal College of Obstetricians and Gynecologists and former chairman of the Department of Obstetrics and Gynecology at the University of Witwatersrand in Johannesburg, South Africa. The development of the decompression birthing bubble took place as a means of unraveling the mysteries of labor, rather than for the purposes of easing childbirth. Nevertheless, it is used effectively now to accomplish the latter.

Dr. Heyns first informed the medical world about the use of abdominal decompression for the first stage of labor in 1959. He wrote: "The effect on the abdominal wall is to make it bulge forward greatly thus allowing the uterus to push forward (become more spherical) without being resisted by a tense abdominal wall . . . There is substantial pain relief in over 90 percent of labours."[2]

What the decompression discoverer suggested was confirmed in 1962 by L. J. Quinn, M.D., and R. A. McKeown, M.D., two American obstetricians. They wrote: "Abdominal decompression is a method of reducing the pain of parturition (childbirth) and of accelerating the first stage of labor. . . . Our latest [studies] confirm our original work and show that this method considerably relieves the pain of labor and shortens the first stage. . . . One of the very important benefits . . . was the ability of so many of the patients to go through labor without any analgesia. This we feel is a very distinct help . . . the babies show no respiratory distress and begin to cry as soon as they are delivered. In our series of 142 patients, 86 (60½ percent) required no analgesia during labor. The remainder required only a small amount . . ."[3]

Abdominal Decompression Reduces the Use of Medication

Hospital obstetrical departments have become accustomed to giving medications. They are naturally reluctant to change from the known benefits of this technique to an unfamiliar one that involves more effort and such an innovative procedure as the use of the decompression birthing bubble. Yet the baby's well-being is a prime consideration. Hospitals are now aware that innovation is worthwhile if it assures the baby the best possible start in life. So long as the infant does fairly well after birth, the difference between excessive sedation and none may seem unimportant. But small problems may appear later, as in the child's speed of learning at school or compatibility with classmates.

Pain-relieving drugs may be necessary during the birth process, at least in small quantities. But if a mother can help her child by using techniques to reduce her need of analgesics as much as possible, the effort is worth it. Now the decompression birthing bubble has come along as another adjunctive technique to reduce the use of medication. It is worth a try. Any mother wants her baby to start life with everything in its favor. She is playing for high stakes—her child's future.

Lois Hyasse Experiences the Baby Bubble

"The night I entered the hospital to give birth to my second daughter there were three people delivering and only one maternity nurse on duty. When the nurse found someone who would do something to assist herself—me—she said, 'Fine, here's a birthing bubble; go ahead and decompress your belly!' I guess she figured we would be there all night. My husband, Arnold, was with me. The doctor wasn't anywhere around.

"The vacuum cleaner sound of that plastic dome enfolding my belly is something I'll never forget. I felt it lift my whole stomach area. At first I was frightened, but then the nurse explained how it was working—lifting the weight off my uterus. I remember very distinctly the words that she used. She said it reduces 'intraamniotic pressure,' and I didn't know if that was good or bad. She told me to push the button on this little switch she had handed me anytime I felt a contraction starting. I did, and the sensation didn't feel bad. I kept pushing the button at the occurrence of each contraction.

"Well, that nurse popped in again and again as I pushed the button with the vacuum machine going on and off. You could hear the noise out in the hall, I guess. Arnold said you could hear it in the next room. The nurse said she couldn't believe that I was setting the machine going only when I was having a contraction. She thought I was playing with it as if the bubble was some kind of toy. I assured her that my contractions really were coming that often. At that time, Arnold and I knew nothing about timing them. I had had no childbirth education. I

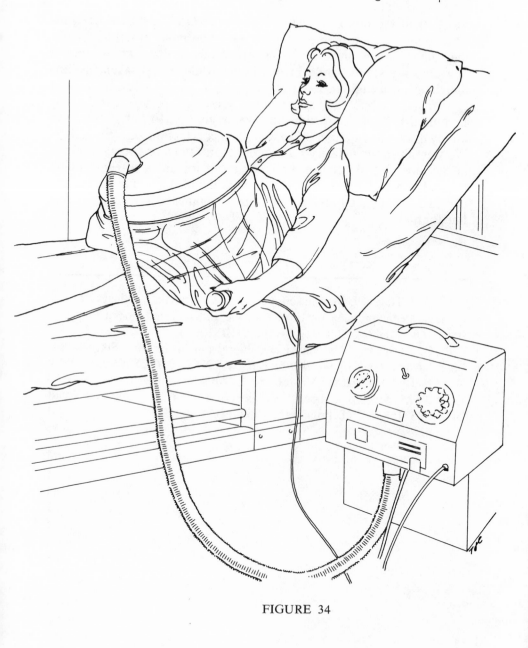

FIGURE 34

just pushed the button whenever that contraction feeling started up. The bubble suction seemed to take away the pain sensation. Maybe the suction effect made my labor go faster—I don't know—but, I delivered my second child in two hours while it had taken my first daughter fourteen hours to come out.

"I found the bubble to be a really interesting experience, and surely I would ask for it again with the next pregnancy. I think it cut down on my discomfort quite a bit so that each contraction was less violent. We weren't in the delivery room more than fifteen or twenty minutes, at the most. I had been in the labor room for about fifteen minutes before the maternity nurse got to me with the birthing bubble, so I had it lifting my stomach area for perhaps an hour and a half. It worked fine for me!"

NOTES FOR CHAPTER FOURTEEN

1. O. S. Heyns, J. M. Samson, and J. A. C. Graham, "Influence of Abdominal Decompression on Intra-amniotic Pressure and Foetal Oxygenation," *The Lancet* I:289–92 (February 10, 1962).

2. O. S. Heyns, "Abdominal Decompression in the First Stage of Labour," *J. Ob.-Gyn. of the British Empire* LXVI: 220–28 (April 1959).

3. L. J. Quinn and R. A. McKeown. "Abdominal Decompression During the First Stage of Labor," *American Journal of Obstetrics and Gynecology* 83:458–63. (February 15, 1962).

15

Leboyer— Birth Without Violence

Creativity redefines the traumatic situations of life by insisting that they are not painful but pleasurable, not destructive but constructive. Thus, we have creative birth, creative firing, creative scarcity, creative marriage and divorce and, to end it all, creative dying. . . . Creative birth introduces the modern child to the world with gentle music and tender smiles rather than a slap on the behind. This new welcome may not be appropriate to life as it is, but it is certainly appropriate to the world many wish to forge. This will be a world that skillfully masks its problems and that anesthetizes the pain they produce with sophisticated rhetoric and elaborately obfuscating philosophies.
—SUZANNE GORDON, The New York Times

The Leboyer Method for Easing the Birth Episode

"Make my baby cry," she pleaded even as the blood gushed from her birth canal where the newborn had been.

"We have a better way now." The maternity nurse smiled behind her mask. "Here we use the Leboyer method for easing the birth episode. Everything is done gently, slowly, softly. Stroke your daughter now and make cooing sounds while I bring over the warm water bath. Baby Johannah is about to return to the water world from which she came."

The childbirth technique of retired obstetrician Frederick Leboyer is based on good common sense—avoid any type of trauma for the newborn. The pushing and pulling at delivery, pressure on the head, loud noises, bright lights shining in the eyes, and the painful sting of slaps on the buttocks are avoided with the Leboyer method. Even holding the infant upside down by the feet to cause the sudden straightening of the spine is not done. Consider that the infant has just arrived from a place where shaping has been with a spine that is curved. The violence of entry into an air-filled world where once there had been only cushioning amniotic fluid can be lessened by not subjecting the baby to noxious stimuli at birth.

Baby Johannah's bond with her mother is being made firmer even while the doctor waits for expulsion of the afterbirth. Placed on her mother's abdomen, the baby feels easy stroking of lightly touching fingers and hears whispered words of love. The bond between them is nurtured in this way. The mother will always remember this feeling and cherish it.

Next comes a soothing bath with water temperature the same as within the womb—98.6 degrees F. Baby Johannah's environment will then be very similar to the one she has just left. The transition to the world of air rather than water will be less traumatic. We do not want to terrify the new being who has come among us.

How Accepted Is the Leboyer Method?

Most obstetricians do offer Leboyer's birth without violence, if you request it in advance. True, there may be a time factor involved. The doctor, busy delivering the placenta or sewing up the episiotomy, may have insufficient opportunity to prepare a bath at just the right temperature and carefully to immerse the infant within it. Dripping blood for fifteen minutes from an unsutured episiotomy would be poor surgical practice. Consequently, an extra helper is required as part of the obstetrical team.

What? You say we are adding to the medical cost? Then let us propose another step forward in Leboyer's childbirth method, one that the developer himself has not used. We recommend assistance by another interested person already in the delivery room—the father.

The father, after having been well-trained during prenatal classes, should be the one to give his baby the warm bath. Daddy will have to be shown how beforehand, of course, and be well-practiced in advance. It is a pleasurable task that he can perform for his newborn and probably will do eventually anyway. Why not firm the paternal bond at the time of birth, as has been accomplished with the maternal bond?

Medical professionals and even home birth proponents who have scoffed at Dr. Leboyer's recommendations have characterized his methods as "birth without parents." They do so because it is only he, the obstetrician, who is shown fondling the newborn. The father, in fact, is never even mentioned by Dr. Leboyer in his writings and lectures. Our suggestion may offset this singular criticism.

The Newborn Responds to the Leboyer Approach

Dr. Leboyer has written a book and produced a film wherein he complains that the advent of birth is not an enjoyable experience for the baby. He writes, "Can birth hold so much suffering, so much pain? While the parents look on in ecstasy, oblivious . . . it's true."

He assures us that the newborn feels everything without choice or discrimination. "Birth is a tidal wave of sensation, surpassing anything we can imagine. A sensory experience so vast we can barely conceive of it."

We agree with each of the techniques that Dr. Leboyer institutes as a means to lighten an infant's burden of birth. We acknowledge that the use of reduced light for delivery, muted sounds, softened wrappings to simulate membranes, and other comfortable components relating to the birth process are important. Entrance into the ambulatory world of sun and air must not be a torture of an innocent being. We would have the parents express love to the baby and begin its journey through life in just this way. We do not adhere to the cynical concepts of Suzanne Gordon with which we began this chapter. Our belief is that the Leboyer approach does provide an infant response with character development that indicates happiness and a feeling of peace with playmates, parents, and self. Dr. Leboyer said:

> What we are doing here is softening the pain of an almost total upheaval by carrying the past forward into the present. We are giving the child company on its journey. We are soothing by sending the echo of the familiar and loving uterine waves along its back. Yes, making love is the sovereign remedy for anguish: to make love is to rediscover peace and harmony. In the cataclysm of birth is it not fit that we should call upon this sovereign comfort?[1]

The Trauma of Being Born

Being born probably is a trauma, caused by the shock of moving from the most comfortable of situations to one where you must make your way in the real world. In your mother's uterus all needs are met—literally a heaven—where no requirement goes unfulfilled and there is nothing else to do except to thrive. When you forsake the comfort of this amniotic cushion for our hard and cold external environment, the experience can be a terrible shock.

Before Frederick Leboyer explored the trauma of typical European and American birth, all of us were shocked into the world in this way. Doctors, midwives, and others pulled us out of our comfortable sacks and beat on our bodies, increasing the trauma of the situation. No wonder that many adults have to undergo psychoanalysis! Fortunately, we know better today.

Obstetrical professionals are now making the new baby's psychological and physical comfort a primary concern by adapting aspects of "birth without violence." They are slowing down the immediate post-delivery process and allowing the baby to adjust at its own speed to life on the outside.

The change to outside living is made smoothly in stages to provide a joyful and happy experience. One way to accomplish this easy transition is to rid the mother of pain and fear connected with childbirth. Previously the infant was affected by her upsetting feelings. Within seconds of life emotional scars were scratched on the child's brain. Such scars have an impact on almost all of us for life.

The Attitude for Birth Without Violence

The procedures for accomplishing birth without violence are performed by the birth attendants in order to minimize the contrasts between the baby's one environment and its next. For this, there is a certain attitude required of the doctor or midwife. No longer is there the incorrect attitude that a baby is a living object that does not see, hear, or have a consciousness. Instead, the little one is treated with the same respect due every human being. He or she has gone through (in most instances) nine months of being created into a whole person, which by itself made a significant impression on the baby's consciousness. In the uterus, he or she felt at ease; arms and legs were folded over; body was somewhat constricted in a bent position; darkness prevailed; it was warm; there was nourishment; no weight of gravity was noticed. As we have described it—heavenly surroundings in which to thrive.

Suddenly there is an extraordinary paroxysm of bumping, squeezing, pushing, and expelling when labor comes on and the child is delivered. Rather than freedom and renewed comfort, which is desired, the new little person is blinded by bright lights, gets his or her spine straightened sharply, is smacked on the behind, is subjected to gravitational pull and density, hears blasts of unfamiliar sounds, feels burned by air as it first fills the lungs, and experiences terror of the unknown. It must be an uncontrollable panic, a total anguish.

Contrasting Procedures of the Leboyer Method

By realizing that a newborn is hypersensitive through the skin, the eyes, the ears, and other senses, it becomes obvious what procedures are taken for the Leboyer method of childbirth. It is a direct contrast to the previous ways of delivery. The baby is delivered in dim light or an indirect light and in silence. Yes, hardly any of the people in the delivery room make sounds. Our observations have been that the noisiest people are not the obstetrical personnel at all but the parents. But who would deny a mother the right to yell if she wishes? Dr. Leboyer suggests that a newborn perceives sounds the same way that a fish does: all over the skin surface. He says, "The whole body is one vast ear."

The newborn is allowed slowly to enter the world of breathing. Air may burn as it first fills the lungs. A little time must pass before the umbilical cord is cut so that the infant has a choice of two ways of breathing. Blood pulses through the cord while the baby takes air from the outside. When pulsation stops the time is ripe for its cutting.

The spine is handled gingerly. No sudden jerks are permitted to uncoil the bent column suddenly, especially no hanging upside down by the feet. This would be brutal treatment only surpassed in cruelty by slapping the baby's body to make him or her cry.

The first touch sensation for the naked infant must be the warm smooth skin of the mother's naked abdomen. The skin-to-skin contact is necessary for permanent maternal-infant attachment, a bonding that will stay with them forever. No cloth wraps or other bedclothes must be put on the baby until much later. Cloth is a foreign substance that may scorch sensitive skin. That first touch must be on the tummy to allow for his or her unfolding from the fetal position slowly, like the petals of a flower. The adoring mother lays her hands along the baby's sides for support, and the father gently strokes the back to supply a feeling of security, the same as it was a few moments before labor contractions struck away the even environment he or she had known for nine months. The parents' hands help to hold him together the way the walls of the uterus had done.[2]

In a little while the newborn will begin to stretch and straighten. The doctor turns the baby on his or her side then and waits until the newborn is quite comfortable before turning him or her on his or her back. Finally, the mother and father prop up their baby in a sitting position with good support. He or she becomes acclimated to the world he or she will live in that way. Only a few minutes have passed for all this. Then the Leboyer bath is used.

The Controversial Water Bath Used by Dr. Leboyer

In the true Leboyer method, a bath is made ready, the water just slightly above body temperature. The newborn is carefully immersed up to the neck to simulate the warm amniotic fluid he or she had been floating in. Dr. Leboyer's thirty-minute film and some photographs in his book show infants with smiles on their faces while they float effortlessly in the one element they are familiar with—warm liquid.

The baby feels weightless again. Pictures show the eyes open, looking all around. The doctor holds the infant under the head at the nape of the neck. The umbilical stub is immersed as well, with no danger of infection considered. Dr. Leboyer says that hot water from the tap is fine, with cold water added as required. One's elbow makes a fine temperature gauge. The baby will play in the bath, moving arms and legs; calmness sets in and crying stops. All this takes from three to six minutes, and an observer will see the tension disappearing from the child. The spine loosens, a smile appears, and the baby waits for what is to come next.

That is the time to dry the infant, dab some antiseptic on the umbilical stump, wrap him or her loosely in soft cotton cloth, and let the mother hold and soothe her baby. The father has a chance to fondle, too.

Dr. Leboyer's water bath is the most controversial of the many techniques he has innovated. We have no objection to it, although others feel alienated by what he recommends and dismiss everything he has had to say. Medical authorities had been upset by what they considered a breach of protocol, since Dr. Leboyer took his findings to the popular press without first publishing them in the medical literature. We believe that his critics are illustrating a classic case of "throwing out the baby with the bathwater."

Some birth authorities think that the baby bath can serve a very useful purpose for the father-infant bonding. It will be an encouragement for the father to participate in the birthing process. All that it would take is the addition of this extra step in the childbirth preparation classes. Dad could practice with a rubber doll and a tub of water

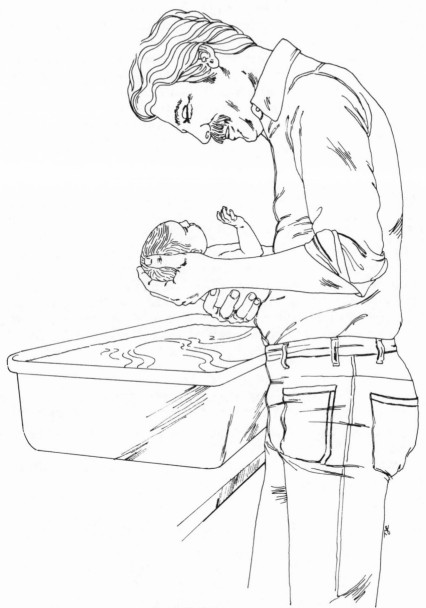

FIGURE 35

adjusted to just the right temperature. By dipping in his elbow along with a thermometer at the same time enables him to know exactly what body temperature water feels like.

One of the young fathers we spoke with who had bathed his daughter right there in the delivery room told us, "Because I gave baby Johannah her bath, I immediately felt totally right in my situation as a new father. I handled my tiny daughter with respect and love, for she was a person in her own right. But she was dependent on me to help her float, and that is how I think it will be from now on. I will help her float through life, giving her support when she wants it and needs it."

Dr. Leboyer's Growing Ranks of Supporters

Dr. Leboyer has developed a method of caring for newborns and their entry into our world. He has a growing number of supporters in the United States. If you desire to join their ranks, write to the Holistic Childbirth Institute, 1627 Tenth Avenue, San Francisco, California 94122. The institute is dedicated to furthering the practice of the Leboyer method of birth without violence. It is one of the "holistic" techniques we shall discuss in Chapter 19.

NOTES FOR CHAPTER FIFTEEN

1. Frederick Leboyer, *Birth Without Violence* (New York: Alfred A. Knopf, 1975).

2. Frederick Leboyer, *Loving Hands* (New York: Alfred A. Knopf, 1976).

16
Maternity Care Focuses on Family Unity

During these months [of pregnancy] I had all the familiar apprehensions about what the baby would be like, but what I dreaded most, I think, was dullness. However, I could do something about anxieties of this kind by disciplining myself not to expect the child to be any special kind of person—of my own devising. I felt deeply—as I still feel—that this is the most important point about bringing into the world a child that will have its own unique and clear identity.
—MARGARET MEAD, *Blackberry Winter: My Earlier Years*

Two Major Parental Attitude Differences

Based on a study conducted by poll takers Yankelovich, Skelly and White, Inc., which explored the problems of raising children in a changing society in 1977, we see that in our society today parents have two distinctly different attitudes about giving birth and family unity.

The *naturalists* in parenting are better educated, more affluent, more permissive with their children, more willing to take risks, believe in the equal rights of children and parents, pursue life-styles that are less child-oriented, question the ideas of sacrificing for children, limit the number of children they have, consider the individuality of a child very important even from the moment of birth, and reject many traditional values.

The *traditionalists* in parenting support values by which they were raised, place considerably more emphasis on strict, old-fashioned upbringing, are convinced that the ways they are familiar with are best, believe in respect for authority, are ready to sacrifice for their children, want their children to be outstanding, lock themselves into the parental disapproval syndrome, possibly feel a suppressed hostility toward their own parents, do not recognize the individuality of a child, think that boys and girls should be raised differently, and are generally private people themselves.

Those who practice natural parenting have many of the values advocated by the college youth of the sixties and seventies. They represent 43 percent of all parents and are less concerned with money and work. Rather they stress family unity and self-fulfillment. The method by which they give birth reflects these feelings. The result is that maternity care has been forced into change to accommodate the new breed of thinking.

Compared to previous generations, new-breed parents regard having children not as a social obligation but as a choice to be made freely and openly. This freedom of choice extends itself to the manner in which they give birth as well. And modern maternity procedures, including orthodox hospital practices, have had to be altered to meet their wishes and demands.

During the weeks surrounding birth, maternity care may be focused on family unity and the closeness of husband, wife, baby, and other members of the immediate family. Family-centered maternity care usually includes the presence of the husband during labor and delivery, and conscious participation of the woman in childbirth. It involves prior education of the couple about pregnancy, childbirth, and breast feeding. The whole family unit is involved, including siblings. Birth may take place in a hospital, at home, or at a childbearing center, but the most important thing is that this is patient-centered care with all members of an immediate family considered the patients.

You have already learned about couple-oriented classes that teach men the art of coaching during labor and delivery. In these classes, the men usually find they like the communication they've shared with their wives and the other couples. They get their doubts and questions answered in an informal setting.

The husband's role is an active and important one among the new breed of parents. He supports his wife physically and psychologically during training and in actual childbearing. The man's coaching participation makes childbirth a total family experience.

Rooming-in for Commencing the Family Unit

In some hospitals, preliminary alterations in their maternity procedures commenced with their allowing the newborn to stay in the room with the mother during her confinement. This practice is called *rooming-in*. It was one of their first recognitions that a new breed of parents was coming on the scene who wanted a firm establishment of the family unit.

Proponents of rooming-in say it is good because baby will be fed on demand. This promotes lactation for breast feeding. A mother's usual anxiety about her infant cradled in another part of the hospital is something the rooming-in parent does not feel. Her infant is in the room all the time. The mother's attention is focused on baby care immediately, and mother and father receive practice for what is going to happen at home when they are on their own. First-time parents learn that baby's demands are not so great—it sleeps almost twenty out of twenty-four hours a day. If the baby has colic, it will be quickly discovered and the pediatrician is on the premises to help.

But there are opponents to rooming-in. They say it is hard on the mother who doesn't feel well after delivery. Arguments are that three, four, or five days are not going to make much difference in learning to be a mother, inasmuch as the baby and the parents will have the rest of their lives to become acquainted in the comfort of their home. Money enters into the picture, too. New parents sometimes are against the idea of paying high costs for postpartum care and then doing all their own work of baby care in the hospital.

Henry L. Harris, M.D., who specializes in infants and children, suggests that there are good and bad points to rooming-in. "Basically it is a good concept because the amount of contact a mother has with her infant from the first day is critical for attachment. The main objection to rooming-in is that not enough experts in baby care get to observe the child in the first twelve to eighteen hours," Dr. Harris said. "Then, many mothers leave the hospital physically exhausted from not coming down from the high excitement caused by the birth. They are superresponsive to the baby's movements, cries, and whimperings. The baby sleeps, but these stimulated mothers don't. Very often the mothers are tuned into the baby too much."

Joan Paspalis, R.N., who works in the newborn nursery at the Stamford (Connecticut) Hospital, thinks that rooming-in should be modified somewhat. The babies should be brought to their mothers throughout the day but carried back to the nursery so the mothers can sleep at night. "It's a very busy time for the new mother who is confined to a hospital room for the first few days. If she kept track of the number of visitors she receives from eight A.M. to nine thirty P.M., I think she would be astounded, what with the physicians, nurses, bookmobile, various volunteers, picture lady, food servers, and guests. All this activity tends to tire her. Sure, we nurses believe that rooming-in is a great idea, an opportunity for a mother to be alone with her baby. Nothing delights me more than to walk in on a young woman who is nestled with her infant in bed, but that is seldom the case. A girl hardly gets time for nestling," said Mrs. Paspalis.

"If a woman ends up socializing and discussing things on the telephone with family and friends, while her baby is lying awake in a crib nearby with no interaction between them, where is the advantage?" asked the pediatric nurse.

One woman described by Nurse Paspalis was quite demanding on the hospital staff and the doctors. She insisted on keeping the baby with her constantly. After three days she looked absolutely exhausted—hardly slept at all. The maternity nurses consulted with the doctor and decided to take the baby out of her room for eight hours without asking her—just told her they were doing it. When they did that, the poor woman broke down and cried in utter relief because somebody had bailed her out. She said, "Thank you, thank you, I am so tired!"

Breast Feeding Becomes a Vital Part of Family-Centered Maternity Care

While bottle feeding today can be as easy as screwing a sterilized nipple onto a bottle of prepared formula that requires no refrigeration until it is opened, maternal preferences are definitely swinging back to the more natural way of child caring. Family-centered maternity care usually includes breast feeding, and there is an increasing number of nursing mothers. Nursing eliminates formula and bottle preparation; however, it requires a more careful diet for the mother and a little more privacy at mealtime for baby. On the other hand, some mothers feel natural enough with the process to nurse the baby in public.

Breast feeding is no either/or proposition. Women with busy schedules or who return to work when the baby is very young, nurse for some meals and bottle-feed for others. Sometimes this alternating method works well, depending on the infant. A baby's demand will determine the supply of breast milk. Before rooming-in, the traditional hospital routines had handicapped breast feeding; but that's no longer the case.

These mothers who make the commitment to breast-feed are prepared to put up with the problems that accompany it. Those problems are not common but they do exist, such as the feeling of inadequacy if the milk flow is poor. When the woman has a poor self-image to start and she finds a problem with her milk supply, her feelings about herself get dashed into the ground even further.

The mother who is nursing well is a contented person. It is a positive cycle. When the baby thrives on her breast milk, the mother feels positive in her response to the baby. The new-breed woman certainly wants that positive feeling. There is more on breast feeding later in the book.

New Childbearing Centers Encourage Family Unity

Mothers-to-be who want to have their babies with their families at their sides but who want to minimize medical risk to themselves and their newborn, can now have the best of both worlds at childbearing centers. Certain hospitals are establishing medical facilities that combine birthing rooms and family living rooms. Together, these rooms combine the physical and psychological comforts of home with instant availability of sophisticated medical equipment and procedures vital to the health of both mother and infant.

At individual childbearing centers around the country, families are viewed along with professionals as active members of the health care team, sharing in decision-making within the limits of safe maternity and infant care. Families are involved as a team at every step of their physical care. Group and individual educational sessions enable the mother and the person she chooses to assist her, to learn and discuss with other parents various aspects of childbearing and parenting in general.

Often there is an informal gathering area where expectant mothers have the freedom to walk around or relax during the early stage of labor.

When active labor begins, the mother and the person she's chosen to be with her (usually the husband-coach) leave the family room and retire to the labor/delivery room.

In childbearing centers, one room serves for both labor and delivery. Furnishings in that room are homelike. Physical care throughout is provided by professionals, and prior to the birthing experience, most parents have a chance to meet and work with all members of the childbearing center's staff. Often the staff is comprised of nurse-midwives.

A Resurgence of Midwifery

A renaissance of the art of midwifery has come upon us since the new mother who thinks as a naturalist has decided to make birthing a family-centered event. Even though birth is the oldest human experience, childbirth in America today is still in the experimental stage for everyone.

Before Queen Victoria's decision to accept chloroform while in labor laid the groundwork for the administration of drugs and the use of hospitals and doctors as the norm in childbirth, midwives delivered almost everyone. For most of human history, attending to childbirth has been woman's work. Billions of babies were helped into the world by lay midwives. By 1910, only 50 percent of American babies were born at home with midwives. Now 90 percent are born in hospitals delivered by physicians.

Some of that is changing. Nurse-midwives are well accepted in many parts of the country and certain medical facilities have them on their staffs. Also lay midwives, while still practicing underground, are attending pregnant women slightly more openly, especially in those more remote areas of the country where there is no available obstetrician. Midwives will help women give birth at home at a saving of nearly $2000 in hospital and obstetrical fees, and the new-breed woman wants that cost saving, as well. Midwifery is discussed in more detail in Chapter 18.

Childbirth at Home Is in the Family-Centered Concept

Some couples have decided, and more are joining the movement every day, that the privacy of their bedrooms provides the most natural setting for a natural birth. Most likely this is where the baby was conceived and, the couples believe, it is where the baby should be born.

Women are in charge of their own deliveries. It is an expression of protest over the way they have been denied control of their own bodies in the past. Skyrocketing prices for American obstetrical care and the very small coverage for maternity costs afforded by medical health insurance are circumstances that also encourage childbirth at home. Childbirth consumerism is spreading. Ten percent of all births in the state of California now take place at home.

Some of these home deliveries are handled by illegal clinics— "underground clinics"—which provide all kinds of counseling services. Not only do they engage in the birth process, they indiscriminately accept young women for abortion. One student nurse-social worker told us she assists in a San Francisco underground obstetrical clinic where she recently counseled a twelve-year-old girl to have an abortion. The student nurse has attended at least three home deliveries and is being taught at the clinic to do pelvic examinations, Pap smears, and almost any other diagnostic procedure a gynecologist performs not requiring certain specialized skill.

Traditionalists Are Influenced by the New Values

While the traditional-minded parents still comprise the majority (57 percent), the attitudes and opinions of the naturalists are having their effect. Traditionalists continue to support the basic values by which they were raised, but they also have been influenced by the new values. There is a reconciliation going on in their minds, a putting together of these changed concepts with older theories and beliefs.

In the next several chapters, we shall discuss in more detail the mechanics of these various modifications in obstetrical procedure that are dedicated so heartily to family-centered maternity care. The decision to take on some of these new ideas may be more difficult for traditional-minded parents, yet, out of fairness, we believe they should have the benefit of knowing more than the basics by which they were raised and the old values to which they subscribe. Maternity care has had to change, and it is likely that other traditionalists will have to change, too.

17

The New "In and Out" Childbearing Centers

Unfortunately, the birthing practices on this continent have become geared to the high-risk case rather than to the normal one. But I believe that the picture is not so gloomy as some critics have charged; you can have the childbirth you choose, within the hospital setting, if you have the tools to work within the system. The tools are information, conviction, tact—and a community which backs you up in your demands.
—VALMAI HOWE ELKINS, *The Rights of the Pregnant Parent*

Adam Sean Walsh Fitzpatrick was born at 11:22 A.M. on a Monday in the New York City Childbearing Center of the Maternity Center Association. Just ten hours later, the jubilant parents, John Fitzpatrick and his wife, Mary, bundled their son into a taxi for the ride home. The baby continued his sleep in the old-fashioned rocking cradle next to his parents' bed.[1]

The Childbearing Center, as it is known, is a specially designed and equipped unit of two birthing rooms installed at the headquarters of the Maternity Center Association. Not in a hospital, the Childbearing Center is staffed by nurse-midwives who are supervised by physicians friendly to the concept of birthing out of the hospital. Each woman who comes to the facility for childbirth is carefully examined and screened for possible medical need and allowed to choose the best method suited to her needs: midwife or obstetrician, hospital or childbearing center or home birth. When indicated, the woman is urged to take hospitalization and more expert obstetrical care to reduce risk of harm to herself or the newborn. Otherwise, the midwives of the Childbearing Center take responsibility for a safe delivery, although they still offer rapid transport, where necessary, to nearby hospitals.

There are a number of such childbearing centers around the country—Eugene, Oregon; Cleveland, Ohio; Albuquerque, New Mexico, and others. About thirty groups belong to an organization called HOME (Home Oriented Maternity Experience) which seek to advance this concept of out-of-hospital childbirth. Surprisingly, even some hospitals featuring "birthing rooms" belong.

The Theory and Practice of Birthing Rooms

Obstetrical preoccupation with the medical and pathological aspects of parturition (giving birth to a child) has reduced perinatal illness and death. But often this preoccupation produces a sterile, dehumanized atmosphere. Birthing rooms in hospitals (and out of them) have come into being to provide both a normal, healthy birth and a creative, joyous experience. Its proper management is an art as well as a science. Therefore, a modern maternity unit should contain a number of private, homelike, fully equipped labor-delivery rooms. These birthing rooms represent a happy compromise between the austerity of the conventional maternity unit and the risks of home delivery. In theory, the plan will individualize and dignify the childbirth experience. In practice, it does work. Birthing rooms have been successful wherever units have been installed.

In these units, the era of twilight sleep and the passive woman in labor is over. New policies are being established to meet the physical and emotional needs of the conscious, active mother-to-be. Most doctors are finally agreeing with feminists who are shouting for respectful attention.

Obstetricians have stepped back and taken a new look at their facilities. They are rearranging their priorities to emphasize the more positive, joyous aspects of childbirth. Frankly, they have had to— parents are demanding it!

Happily, homelike labor-delivery rooms are working exceedingly well. As an illustration, Martin L. Stone, M.D., professor and chairman of the Department of Obstetrics and Gynecology at New York Medical College, Flower and Fifth Avenue Hospitals, in New York City, described his facility's "Family Living Room": "In the hospital living room, the mother can be as relaxed as she would be if she were having her baby at home. During her labor period, she may sit up in an easy chair or lie in bed, watch TV, read, chat with her husband or other relative or friend she has chosen to share the adventure of birth with."

What Typical Birthing Rooms Look Like

The Memorial Hospital in Phoenix, Arizona, accommodates prospective parents with birthing rooms. They are a cheerful two-room suite, and the combination labor-delivery room has walls that are bright with yellow and brown sunflowers. The bed is covered with a gay quilted spread and a nearby lamp, with a colorful Mexican pottery base, gives off a soft glow in the room. The second part of the suite is a living room with sofa, chairs, and a television set, complete with a bean bag chair for the mother. In between the two rooms is a viewing window with curtains that may be drawn. If both mother and doctor agree, observers may look through the window or even be present in the bedroom itself during delivery.

"We decided to recreate the home environment within the hospital and to eliminate the need for an overnight stay," said Reginald Ballantyne 3d, the hospital president. "The demand is unbelievable. We're going to have to add another." The birthing rooms were installed at the Memorial Hospital on September 1, 1976.

"There was a swelling of interest in home deliveries," Mr. Ballantyne said, "and we were concerned that home deliveries may not be in the best interest of good patient care."[2]

Similarly, the New York Medical College, Flower and Fifth Avenue Hospitals' family living room has a rocking chair, an upholstered comfortable chair, and a television set. A small wall light casts a warm glow on the cream-and-gold-striped wallpaper, the purple cottage curtains, and a hanging flowerpot. Books and magazines fill a black-walnut-stained hutch. Dr. Stone shopped for the furnishings himself.

In the next room an ordinary-looking bed stands ready for birthing. It has all the trappings necessary for delivery of babies, including a large overhead tilted mirror at its foot.

These various birthing rooms were established out of a conviction that in-hospital maternity care should be as compassionate, personalized, and family-centered as possible within standards of safety. The events surrounding the birth of a child should be an emotionally satisfying experience for all members of the family to contribute to the development of a healthy family unit.

The Family Is Part of the Health Care Team

"The siblings are involved now when the parents want them to be," said Ruth Watson Lubic, R.N., CNB, general director of the Maternity Center Association (MCA).

"They witness the birth of their new brother or sister, if the parents desire that. We have no objection."

Since 1970, the MCA had been alerting professionals and the public to the growing trend among young mothers and families to seek alternatives to high hospital costs and traditional systems of maternity care. Reports from around the nation revealed that a growing number of couples were turning to unsupervised home delivery. The MCA subsequently set up an experimental demonstration project in New York City based on the obstetrician/nurse-midwife team concept. It was designed to offer a homelike setting that is safe, satisfying, and low-cost.

The candidates for childbearing at the MCA center must be considered low risk: A woman giving birth for the first time can be no older than thirty-five; a woman who's had up to four children can be no older than thirty-nine—if she has had more than four children and is age thirty-nine, she is atuomatically ineligible; a history of three or more miscarriages is a barrier. There is no minimum age requirement, and the youngest patient delivered was sixteen. The MCA childbearing service fee is $750 for everything, including prenatal care, use of the birthing rooms, nurse-midwife delivery, and postpartum care.

Obviously, the MCA Childbearing Center operates with rigid rules on the mother's physical condition for safety, but it allows enormous latitude in procedures. One family, for example, as the MCA director pointed out, was permitted to have its two-year-old son in the delivery room while the mother gave birth.

"We are trying to provide an alternative for the alternative of home delivery," Ruth Lubic told us. It is something safer than do-it-yourself, and yet provides people with the kind of emotional support that they feel at home. It is the sense that the family is together, the triad of the couple, the new infant, and the siblings.

"This doesn't mean that the family tells the nurse-midwife or the obstetrician what to do, but it does mean that the family is part of the decision-making body. The family is informed of the options and they decide on the kind of experience they desire in this unit. If a woman wants an all-fours birthing position, something not customary in our culture, we will do everything in our power to accommodate her," Mrs. Lubic said. "In effect, we work at making the family an integral part of the health care team."

In addition to giving couples as much control as possible over the delivery of their children, the MCA Childbearing Center propounds other medical purposes:

- To demonstrate that low-risk pregnancies and deliveries need not be treated in a traditional hospital setting.
- To eliminate, when appropriate, such routine procedures as strapping mothers to tables and immobilizing their legs in stirrups, and administering enemas, pubic shaves, and episiotomies.
- To allow parents and babies to remain together for the entire stay and permit them to go home within twelve hours.

"We don't see this as the right unit for every woman," said Mrs. Lubic. "What we're interested in is offering options and alternatives. We didn't set ourselves up just as an alternative to hospitals but to bring back into the system those families who had lost trust and refused to go to the hospital."

The Key Word Is "Trust"

In 1969 Manchester Memorial Hospital, Manchester, Connecticut, established a "Lamaze labor-delivery room" in which the woman who was trained in psychoprophylaxis would both labor and deliver. The program has been successful and is continuing. The monitrice (an obstetrical nurse specifically trained in the Lamaze method) has the responsibility of running the room and providing uninterrupted support to the new parents. She acts similar to a private duty nurse in that her sole responsibility is to the one pregnant patient; she is called when needed and remains with the two parents until one hour postpartum. She bills them directly for her services and is not a hospital employee.

This monitrice concept is useful to assure continuous, knowledgeable, one-to-one support and promotes intuitive trust on the part of both parents. Acting as a skilled labor coach, the monitrice usually is a childbirth educator, certified by the American Society for Psychoprophylaxis in Obstetrics (ASPO).

From its inception until 1976, a total of sixteen hundred maternity patients have been managed with desirable results in this special Manchester Memorial Hospital room. Medication and anesthesia were used selectively for some mothers, but only when absolutely indicated.

Infection is no problem. There is an exceedingly low incidence of complications. The Lamaze labor-delivery room continues to get active use, since the program has been accepted with great enthusiasm both by patients and obstetrical personnel.[3]

In such a program families know that they can have confidence in the in-hospital situation. The wishes of the patient and her mate are respected, and they have a knowledgeable consumer advocate in their monitrice. Occasionally childbirth requires medical or surgical intervention, and for this reason hospital delivery is mandatory.

While some may argue that childbirth at home offers more joyous and meaningful surroundings, it may not provide adequate medical safety in the event of complication. The best maternity unit—one coming into use more often—offers medical safety *and* emotionally comfortable surroundings. This will engender the necessary trust between patients and their professional helpers. "In and out" birthing facilities that are part of or have access to hospitals seem to fulfill these qualifications.

People Who Enjoyed "In and Out" Home-Style Delivery

Where tiny Brinca Johnson was born, in Phoenix's Memorial Hospital, it was a far cry from the glaring lights and sterile atmosphere of the traditional hospital delivery room. Brinca's three-year-old sister, Jamie, watched her entry into the world. And not only did her father come along to bring Jamie, but he also brought a neighbor and the neighbor's own two children, three-year-old Sarah and twelve-year-old Amy Blackburn. There was a regular crowd around to cheer Brinca's exit from her mother's body.

"I'm going to have a baby, too," young Jamie said later, and "all my children will watch." Her mother, Janice Johnson, nodded and smiled.

The people who have "in and out" home-style delivery like the Johnson family usually enjoy satisfying experiences. They are not at the mercy of a method. They are more able to retain control of their situation and can get through it with dignity and a sense of accomplishment.

In some "in and out" childbearing centers the husbands may even be welcome to lie on the labor bed with their wives. One family at the MCA Childbearing Center had the husband sitting with his back against the head of the bed, legs spread wide apart while the wife sat between his legs. She would lie back against him between contractions. When she felt a new contraction coming she squeezed his hand, and he then would help her sit upright and apply pressure to her lower back where she felt severe labor pain. His counterpressure relieved her physical discomfort, and the body contact was emotionally reassuring for both of them.

Lillian and Richard Frey arrived at the Flower and Fifth Avenue Hospitals a few minutes after midnight, long after Mrs. Frey's labor pains had begun. Six weeks of prenatal education had prepared them for what to expect. They were not thrown by the first labor pain. At about 1:20 A.M. Mrs. Frey climbed into the birthing bed after her obstetrician, Dr. Martin Stone, told her it was time. Half an hour later, Mr. and Mrs. Frey shared the exhilarating experience of witnessing the birth of their eight-pound daughter.

Mrs. Frey recalls that her husband "really enjoyed it. He talked all the way through. It was easy and relaxed with him there. I don't think I could have done it without him," she said.

For Mrs. Joanne Cain, the appeal of the birthing room at Memorial Hospital in Phoenix included the opportunity to have her five-year-old daughter, Joleen, participate in the birth. Mrs. Cain spent nine months preparing her daughter for the birthing event and asked her sister, Jean Robertson, to accompany Joleen.

The little girl was ready for the birth, but her aunt was not.

"I faint really easy," Mrs. Robertson said, "and we had to leave the room. My head started to get light. The baby was born right after we walked out of the room."

Joleen returned to enjoy the experience and was the first one to hold her new brother.

Rebecca Pollack and Vincenza Garcia Chose the MCA Childbearing Center

Rebecca Pollack and Vincenza Garcia described the reasons that had brought them to the Childbearing Center of the Maternity Center Association.

Mrs. Pollack said that originally she had been unable to decide between a home or hospital delivery. "I've never felt comfortable even visiting a hospital," she explained, "and I was sure it would be better for me in a setting where I felt at home and more in charge of things, instead of having to put up with all sorts of rules and formalities."

In addition, Mr. and Mrs. Pollack planned to follow the "gentle" method of childbirth—the Leboyer Method—and this increased their reluctance to choose traditional hospital care. They were going to have their baby at home.

However, they were unable to find a physician who agreed to attend a home delivery. After inquiring at a number of hospitals, they were in a dilemma. It was at this point that Mrs. Pollack read a press report of the Childbearing Center—"and I came running," she said.

Vincenza Garcia had a similar experience. She, too, had asked about maternity care at a number of hospitals. "The impression I had," she said, "was that I was being treated like someone with an illness, instead of someone who was simply having a baby. And they didn't give me any real sense of support or preparation."

At the Childbearing Center, she said, "From the time I walked in, I felt that I was receiving support, and I gained confidence in myself, so that not only could I have the baby, but I could take him home immediately afterward and be a responsible parent."

Families at the center learn to respect their own judgment, Mrs. Garcia noted, "because the staff encourages you to do that. With medical guidance, you feel that you can handle the situation."

Care at the MCA Childbearing Center is provided by a team of obstetricians and nurse-midwives, assisted by a pediatrician and the Visiting Nurse Service of New York, which offers follow-up care at home in the first days after birth. Families return to the center for examination seven days after delivery and again in the sixth postpartum week.

Mrs. Pollack had an adverse reaction to this team approach at first, but her apprehension soon faded, she said. "What I found was that I was learning a great deal more, because each nurse-midwife has a special area of interest—in nutrition, exercise, and so on. As time passed I became very pleased with how much I was learning, and in that sense it was even more valuable."

She added that, from the moment her daughter was born, her husband "has been as comfortable with her as I am, and as much her father as I am her mother. Naturally, that's been a delight to her and to me, too," said Mrs. Pollack.

NOTES FOR CHAPTER SEVENTEEN

1. Nadine Brozan, "New Childbirth Center: Baby Born in Morning Was Home by Evening," *The New York Times,* March 27, 1976.

2. Athia Hardt, "In Phoenix Hospital, Birthing Room Offers Home-Style Delivery," *The New York Times,* July 12, 1977.

3. Philip E. Sumner, John P. Wheeler, and Samuel G. Smith, "The Home-like Labor-Delivery Room," *Connecticut Medicine* 40:319–22 (May 1976).

18

Midwifery Services, Both Certified and Underground

> Midwifery-managed pregnancies and deliveries
> have become, almost overnight, a real alternative
> to the usual birth experience for women who are
> in a position to choose the kind of care they
> want. We are no longer serving only to relieve the
> doctors of an overwhelming load of clinic
> deliveries; rather, we offer a unique option for
> women who want to have an increased
> participation in the birth of their children.
> —BARBARA BRENNAN, C.N.M. (and Joan
> Rattner Heilman), *The Complete Book of
> Midwifery*

Current Status of the Nurse-Midwife Profession

The modern nurse-midwife is not one of those old "grannies" who used to ride the back roads on horseback, delivering babies. They don't chew tobacco, all wash their hands before approaching the woman in labor, and none is likely to advocate a big dose of castor oil after delivery or call for a knife under the pillow and an ax under the bed "to cut the pain"—as was the superstition in years gone by.

The current status of the nurse-midwife profession is much changed from the time of the unhygienic, toothless granny. Although there is a recognized old midwife tradition in the United States, today's nurse-midwives are highly trained professionals skilled in the management of normal pregnancy, labor, and delivery, as well as postpartum care and care of the newborn. Their orientation is on childbirth as a natural phenomenon while avoiding any unnecessary interference in the birth process.

Nurse-midwife services are represented nationally by the American College of Nurse-Midwives (ACNM), 1000 Vermont Avenue, NW, Washington, D.C. 20005. Telephone: (202) 628-4642. For information about a nurse-midwife clinic or other professional birth services supplied by trained midwives near you, contact the ACNM.

The modern nurse-midwife must hold a registered nurse degree, to which she adds at least one year of additional clinical experience in maternity care and delivery. She is then qualified to take the nurse-midwife examination given by the ACNM. Only when she passes that does she become a Certified Nurse-Midwife (C.N.M.), accepted by the American College of Obstetricians and Gynecologists as a specialist empowered to assume responsibility for the complete care of uncomplicated maternity patients. However, she still does not function alone but rather as a part of a medically directed team. All of the midwifery-training programs in the United States (eighteen at the last count), emphasize that any aspect of obstetrical care may be handled by the midwife as long as the pregnancy is normal.

Consequently, the certified nurse-midwife is not an independent practitioner. She is usually affiliated with a health institution and has access to the resources of that institution, including the ability to consult with an obstetrician. Such a consultation results in the physician taking on the responsibility for that patient. The nurse-midwife continues to administer to the patient's needs but under the supervision of the doctor she has called in.

How Nurse Midwifery Differs from Lay Midwifery

We have indicated that the certified nurse-midwife is a professional nurse with added specialized knowledge and skill gained through an organized program of study and clinical experience. Working with the physician, the nurse-midwife is prepared to manage and provide care to mother and baby throughout the maternity cycle as long as progress is normal. In contrast, the lay midwife has no professional training and most often is scorned by physicians. She takes no examination, is not certified, and gets her education on the job, usually apprenticing with another lay midwife.

Few women would question the advantage of having another woman attend her at childbirth, yet obstetrical nursing fails to attract a substantial number of recruits because specializing in this area is not as professionally rewarding. Our inquiries of several obstetrical (Ob) nurses lead us to believe that they feel defeated as nurses when they are unable to give expectant mothers the comfort and support they need, or when the Ob nurses are called upon to perform professional tasks for which they feel inadequate.

On the other hand, Jean Cranch, C.N.M, who is assistant director of the Childbearing Center of the Maternity Center Association, told us, "The nurse-midwife tries to orchestrate the kind of birthing a mother wants. Her job is one of monitoring the mother's safety and to give support where it is needed." That is how nurse-midwifery differs from obstetrical nursing but that is not how it differs from lay-midwifery.

Lay midwives are illegal in many states, and they perform their services from an underground network with referrals accepted only from people they know. Still, it is impossible to look at the whole birth catalog of alternatives today without being aware of the return of the lay midwife. She is a modern, talented version of the compassionate old granny.

The underground movement for illegal midwifery is swelling because of a renewed demand among new-breed parents for home birth and among women in general to take control of their own bodies.

As we have said, the women who deliver babies in the home are independent workers with no medical training and no institutional affiliation. Instead, they apprentice under the guidance of another, more experienced lay midwife or they just render birthing assistance that may come instinctively to any woman. They assist as birthing attendants because they are needed and wanted.

A famous lay midwife, Ina May Gaskin, head midwife at The Farm, a large-scale homesteading community in Summertown, Tennessee, who has participated in over seven hundred births, admitted that she got into midwifery out of necessity and without training. Ina May said, "We have become a community and we were on the road, and we couldn't go back to the way it had been before when we lived separately and didn't take care of one another. Some ladies started having babies, and then we met a doctor who had heard we'd delivered two babies and wanted to help us. Since we were delivering our own babies, he questioned whether we knew everything that was required to provide good care for the mother. And he gave us a free lesson in obstetrics. I called him on the phone a couple of times after we got to Tennessee, and he continued to help us at that level."[1]

Lay midwives usually assist at births more as an avocation rather than as a money-making occupation. They feel a strong "calling" to protect and support the birthing woman and her family. Lay midwives consider their presence as the alternative to impersonal hospitals, medication, and infant-parent separation. Their fees, if charged at all, are very low—perhaps $200 for all care. They believe that the eventual licensing and recognition of lay midwives will be part of the forward march of medical science.

Although there are male midwives most midwives are women—mothers themselves. Midwives, both certified and underground, are increasing the public's sensitivity to birthing practices and making professionals in health care think as consumers as well as providers.

Midwife Philosophy Fits Today's Young Parents

Ruth T. Wilf, Ph.D., a certified nurse-midwife at Booth Maternity Center, Philadelphia, and a staff member of Jefferson Medical College, espoused the philosophy of the nurse-midwife when she addressed the 1977 annual conference of the National Association of Parents and Professionals for Safe Alternatives in Childbirth (NAPSAC, Inc.).

Dr. Wilf said, "Having a baby should not only be safe medically, but also a time of personal growth and strengthening for all family members through the creation of an environment which supports human enrichment. This is basically, of course, what we call family-centered maternity care and involves childbirth preparation and support, participation of family members, a conscious birth—usually with direct participation—immediate and extended contact with the newborn to promote parent-infant attachment, and help with breast feeding, infant care and new parenting.

"The entire experience is viewed as a positive part of living," Dr. Wilf explained, "with emphasis on fostering a sense of achievement, good interpersonal relations, and building bonds with the baby."[2]

Accordingly, the American College of Nurse-Midwives adopted the following resolutions:

> Every childbearing family has a right to a safe, satisfying maternity experience with respect for human dignity and worth; for variety in cultural forms; and for the parents' right to self-determination.

> Comprehensive maternity care, including education and emotional support as well as management of physical care throughout the childbearing years, is a major means for intercession into, and improvement and maintenance of, the health of the nation's families. Comprehensive maternity care is most effectively and efficiently delivered by interdependent health disciplines.

Nurse-Midwifery is an interdependent health discipline focusing on the family and exhibiting responsibility for insuring that its practitioners are provided with excellence in preparation and that those practitioners demonstrate professional behavior in keeping with these stated beliefs.[3]

Thus, the ACNM has thoroughly emphasized the interdisciplinary team concept with a strong, binding commitment that in this country a certified nurse-midwife always functions within the framework of a regional or local health service with qualified medical direction. That philosophy tends to eliminate the nurse-midwife from closing sisterly ranks with the lay midwife.

The Legal Status of Lay Midwives in America

The certified nurse-midwife has qualifying standards that reassures the pregnant woman of her competence. Certification is predicated on her taking responsibility for the labor and delivery only when they are normal. But a lay midwife has no qualifying standards. There is no certification test for her. How can you determine whether she is competent and qualified to attend you? Ina May Gaskin says, "I guess you'd have to ask all of your deepest questions, look deep in her eyes and see whether she is somebody you can trust. You just have to use your good judgment."[4]

The legal status of lay midwives in most states in America is in question. They perform their childbirth functions under jeopardy of being arrested for practicing medicine without a license. Therefore the courts are likely to contend that any nonphysician or nonlicensed midwife who presents herself or himself as an expert in labor and delivery and attends a childbirth is guilty of that crime. The California Supreme Court recently ruled that the California legislature has an "interest in regulating the qualifications of those who hold themselves out as childbirth attendants . . . for many women must necessarily rely on those with qualifications which they cannot personally verify."[5] The state of California in this way determines who may receive a license to deliver the babies of its citizens.

Not only that, parents who have a lay midwife assist in home birth may be putting themselves in jeopardy as well. Parents do not have to safeguard their fetuses according to state law, but they do have to protect the newborn. If they don't, they can be prosecuted for child abuse. An aggressive prosecutor may consider that the presence of a lay midwife at childbirth constitutes child abuse if the parents had suspicioned that complications were likely that resulted in permanent injury or death of the child. In fact, if the death was foreseeable, the charge could be manslaughter.[6]

How Lay Midwives Are Attempting to Change Their Legal Status

On November 30, 1977, the legal ban on the licensing of lay midwives by the state of Illinois was upheld by the Federal District Court for the Northern Division of Illinois. The suit was brought by ten women who wanted to be licensed lay midwives, plus twenty parents who contended that they should have the constitutional right to have lay midwives deliver their babies at home. That was the first legal challenge of the laws on midwifery. Fourteen other states, most of them in the South, now license lay midwives. Warren Pease, M.D., of the American College of Obstetricians and Gynecologists, said in a position paper that the World Health Organization had recommended that midwives have three years of formal training, including a year of nursing. "These are the standards being adopted in the developing countries of Nigeria and New Guinea," he said. "Why should the U.S. accept less?"[7]

With about 250 lay midwives in the State of California attending annually to approximately twelve thousand home births, a training and licensing bill has been introduced into the legislature by two assemblymen—Gary Hart and John Vasconcellos. The bill was written by the state's Department of Community Affairs, which protects consumers from fraud and tries to act in their interest. It is designed to go into effect sometime in 1979 and could set an important precedent for the legal status of lay midwives in the nation at large. This fact makes the California legislature's reaction to the bill vital to the growth and popular use of lay midwifery throughout the United States.

The bill, AV-1896, would permit a midwife to manage and care for the mother and her newborn during the prenatal, interpartum, and postpartum stages of normal childbirth. As an independent practitioner, the lay midwife would not act under the aegis of a supervising health agency as do nurse-midwives. She could practice solo like any physician. Her training would take place in a clinical setting as an apprentice to professionals, including scholastic study. She would take training with a physician, nurse-midwife, or a certified lay midwife who has gone through the training before. That way the lay midwife might become a professional. It could take up to two years to achieve certification.

After that, the certified lay midwife would be required by law to get the advice of a licensed physician whenever any childbirth problems arose. Consultation could be by telephone alone. The bill would permit lay midwives to attend pregnant women in outlying areas away from hospital facilities to help overcome the maldistribution of medical services in this country.

However, Bill AV-1896 is being opposed by the California Medical Association, the California Nursing Association, and the California Board of Hospitals.

Services Supplied by Nurse-Midwives and Some Lay Midwives

The services supplied by midwives may vary, depending on whether they are trained or not. Some lay midwives have taken the trouble to learn about perinatal and postnatal procedures. In serving women in more remote areas, these lay midwives probably provide a full prenatal program, including the usual medical care with several hour-long visits. The visits are devoted to taking a complete history; a physical examination within the midwife's realm of capability; a pelvic exam, pelvimetry, and laboratory work; lots of discussion about prenatal nutrition; the standard monthly checkups until the eighth month, then bimonthly, then weekly until labor.

Educated lay midwives encourage people to participate actively in their own care, checking their own urine, weight, and blood pressure, learning as much as possible about pregnancy and the birth process. If the lay midwife is concerned but unskilled in the prenatal procedure, she will usually refer her patient to a friendly physician who offers the prenatal care necessary.

The certified nurse-midwife provides prenatal care in conjunction with an obstetrician, who normally conducts the initial examination, including the usual history, physical, and laboratory work. At subsequent office visits, the mother-to-be may see the same nurse-midwife or another of a rotating group who provide information and answer questions in all areas of obstetrical science. Frequently there are childbirth education classes offered by the institution employing the nurse-midwife, and she makes herself available to answer questions that may arise as a result of the parents attending those classes.

During labor, a lay midwife will probably sit with the mother throughout the process and then deliver the baby. For birthing in the home, a lay midwife most likely will arrive with a few other support people in the event a complication requires that the mother be carried out for transportation to a hospital. The lay midwife makes it a personal rule not to depend on the woman's husband, who might become too excited or upset to be useful in time of crisis. For a nurse-midwife, that is not the required practice. An obstetrician is in or nearby the health institution with which she is affiliated.

Both kinds of midwives attempt to provide a nurturing, noninterfering environment according to the wishes of the parents and modified according to their medical need. The nurse-midwife, of course, is restricted somewhat by the rules of the hospital in which she works. Both midwives give follow-up care during postnatal visits. Following the nurse-midwife's service, the visiting nurse association may make home visits to the mother and child, while the lay midwife pays her own house calls.

In summary, midwives in America are drawing on traditions established by the old-time grannies, the pioneers who carved our cities out of the wilderness. Today's midwives are actively seeking sound medical knowledge to blend with their intuitive understanding of birth, life, and death. Many lay midwives want to be legalized so as not to come into conflict with the medical mainstream. Both kinds of midwives, legal and not, are constantly questioning established birthing patterns and draw from within themselves integral teaching and healing skills. Rather than replacing old patterns with personal beliefs, they are providing the environment for parents to explore the meaning of birth in their own lives.

Certified nurse-midwives have bonded themselves together in a professional organization to provide a much needed service for their communities. In early 1977 lay midwives attempted to do the same but without success. They wanted to cooperate with each other and they could not. Perhaps there will come a time when all midwives will work jointly and in harmony with encouragement from the medical community at large to advance obstetrical science even further than it has come. Mothers and their newborns will be the winners then.

NOTES FOR CHAPTER EIGHTEEN

1. Peggy Taylor, "Ina May, Life and Birth on the Farm," *New Age* 3: 43–5 (October, 1977).

2. Ruth T. Wilf, "Fulfilling the Needs of Families in a Hospital Setting: Can It Be Done?" in *21st Century Obstetrics Now!* ed. Lee Stewart and David Stewart. (Chapel Hill, N.C.: The National Association of Parents and Professionals for Safe Alternatives in Childbirth, 1977).

3. Philosophy of the American College of Nurse-Midwives, 1000 Vermont Avenue, NW, Washington, D.C. 20005, April 22, 1972.

4. Taylor, "Ina May."

5. *Bowland* v. *Municipal Ct. for Santa Cruz City,* 134 Cal. 630, 638

(1976). See also *Magit* v. *Board of Medical Examiners*, 366 P. 2d 816 (Cal. 1961); *Sanfilippo* v. *State Farm Mutual Automobile Ins. Co.*, 535 P. 2d 38 (Arizona 1975).

6. See *State* v. *Sheperd*, 255 Iowa 1218 (1973) and discussion in J. Robertson, "Involuntary Euthanasia of Defective Newborns: A Legal Analysis," *27 Stanford Law Review* 213 (1975).

7. "Ban on Licensing of Lay Midwives Is Upheld by U.S. Judge in Illinois," *The New York Times,* November 30, 1977.

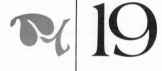

19

The Rebirth of Childbirth at Home

Giving birth has the inherent duality of being at once unique to each woman and universal to all women. The experience divides and unites us. I think it would divide us less, were more women to understand that its simple yet intricate natural process can give a new dimension to the quality of life. I have seen childbirth mark the transition of girl to woman. If the transition is to be complete, the creative aspect of the receptive function must be understood. In accepting receptivity, we become creative.
—DANAË BROOK, *Naturebirth*

The Rebirth of Home Birth

We spoke with new-breed parents Harry and Sally Anderson about their two babies that were born at home and how it was handled effectively.

"God willing, if we have more children, I won't consider having them any other way except at home," said Sally. "I gave birth in my own bed aided by Harry and my lay midwife in the presence of my mother and father, three sisters and brother, and their spouses. It was wonderful to have all that support. Their love just washed over me and lifted me. I feel good about it—very fulfilled. My body and mind are relaxed and comfortable even though I worked hard."

Harry said, "She was just great all the way. The breathing and muscle control exercises she had practiced certainly paid off. Only once or twice did I have to remind her to take a deep cleansing breath before and after contractions. The transition phase lasted only three minutes. Sally made up her own pattern of breathing. There was no hyperventilation, so that after the delivery her body was totally at ease. The perineum stretched by itself with no tearing of tissue—no episiotomy needed—no calling on any doc to sew her up."

"As far as the baby is concerned," Sally said, "she's as keen and alert this morning as a five-day-old. She was this way even immediately at birth, and I can compare her to the others. She's my fifth, you know. When I nursed her a few minutes ago little Harriet was so eager; it made me feel that I did the right thing for her, for me, and for my other loved ones. Harriet's sisters and brothers know all about having babies now. They saw their sister being born."

"Assisting the midwife in the birth of my baby girl was one of the greatest experiences of my life," added Harry. "I only hope I'll be able to experience it again. Sally and I want a dozen children, and all the rest of them can be born at home if my wife wants it that way. Though I love all five of my children equally, the last two, born with Sally sitting up in our marriage bed, are the ones I shall always feel closest to." Harry bent down and kissed his wife.

Sally concluded: "Oh, I know that I was one of the lucky ones to have such easy pregnancies and deliveries, so it's tough for me to tell other women that having your baby at home would be best for them. Not every woman might be as decided as I was. I am completely sold on having labor and delivery—the whole thing—take place at home."

Harry and Sally Anderson are representative of the new breed of parents who have given rebirth to the popularity of home birth. In the years from 1972 to 1975, a time when total births in the United States declined, the number of home births burgeoned by 60 percent. From the beginning of 1976 to the end of 1977, the monthly incidence of home births increased by twenty times, according to home birth educators of the Association for Childbirth at Home, International (ACHI).

A group of Chicago physicians has organized the American College of Home Obstetrics (ACHO). And various home birth groups of laypersons have formed in many U.S. cities such as Seattle, Boston, and Takoma Park, Maryland. In Toronto, SACH (Safe Alternative Childbirth at Home) has been created, which is analogous to the American organization called HOME (Home Oriented Maternity Experience) that we had mentioned in Chapter 17. In Chapel Hill, North Carolina, the National Association of Parents and Professionals for Safe Alternatives in Childbirth (NAPSAC) is holding national conferences and publishing its own books about home birth.

All this activity means that every couple, naturalists or traditionalists, owe it to themselves and their baby to study what options are available in their community and then choose the manner of childbirth that best suits them. Ideally, the couple will have read educational material on birthing and its many ramifications, made the necessary preparations months in advance of the baby's due date, and selected the way they will have their baby from the vast catalog of alternatives available.

Home Birth Is the Practice of Holistic Medicine

There is a growing consciousness throughout the land that says each individual must take responsibility for his or her own health. This kind of thinking is called *holism*, a word derived from the Greek *holo* meaning both *holy* and *whole*. Persons who view themselves holistically take into account every available concept and skill for their growth toward harmony and balance. It means treating the *person*, not a *disease*. It means using mild, natural methods whenever possible and living life to its fullest and healthiest. The holistic approach promotes the interrelationship and unity of body, mind, and spirit. It encourages healthy, enjoyable activity on all these levels of existence.

Home birth is a part of holistic medicine. Indeed, another of the myriad organizations created, this time in San Francisco, is the Holistic Child Movement group. The home birth holistic movement focuses on birth attendants being present but not performing their services unless called upon by necessity. The father and mother perform the birthing of their own child. It takes courage and much education to take responsibility not only for one's own health but also for the health of the newborn.

Recommendations Before Engaging in Birthing at Home

Advance planning makes the difference between a successful home delivery and one that just happens. Many engaged in natural parenting have stressed this point to us. Admittedly, we are not oriented to childbirth at home, but we do defend the right of couples to elect this manner of birthing. Here we provide information about the process, gleaned from home birth educators whom we have interviewed.

There are some considerations that you should take into account before venturing into home birth. First, you should read all the educational material on birth you can get; we have included information sources in the appendices. Then you should have routine prenatal attention for determining that no specialized care for mother or child is required and to have standby arrangements in case emergency assistance is needed during the delivery. Approach the use of obstetrical techniques with caution and care. These are important considerations before engaging in your own birthing at home.

Obstetrical technique is gotten from two sources: medical textbooks and people who deliver babies. Perhaps you have declared yourself determined to have a home birth—O.K.—but you should see an obsetrician to make sure it is a reasonable thing for you to do, both physically and emotionally. There must be no foreseeable complications. Ask the doctor how to deliver yourself or how your husband should deliver you. If you are fortunate to have found a capable midwife or other birth attendant, you should ask that person to assist —at least with verbal instructions, if not actively. Perhaps the physician will agree to participate in assisting your home delivery.

The American College of Home Obstetrics (ACHO)

The American College of Home Obstetrics (ACHO) was founded by its current president, Gregory J. White, M.D., author of the book, *Emergency Childbirth*. Dr. White is also a founding father of the La Leche League International, which we shall describe in the next chapter.

ACHO joins together a number of physicians across the country who wish to cooperate with families who are giving birth at home. ACHO physician members dedicate themselves to learning and teaching each other the "art of the safe supervision of home births," and they foster the welfare of not only mother and baby, but the whole family as a unit.

Dr. White explained that home-birth physicians do not bring a nurse to the home as an assistant but go it alone in the supervisory capacity. The physicians, in fact, do not deliver the infant; they let the parents perform the birth of their own baby. "The important thing," said Dr. White, "is to try to restrain oneself from interfering in a way that would either decrease safety or diminish joy and the full participation of the couple who are 'doing their thing.' I have had more problems with this than the younger doctors, because I had some obstetric training. I think on the whole we have been pretty successful in avoiding any unnecessary interferences.

"But I still think that a professional attendant who knows what he or she is doing, and who is willing to sort of fade into the wallpaper and let the couple do their thing, as long as everything is going well, is still the ideal for delivery at home or anywhere else," said Dr. White.[1]

For information about an ACHO physician member coming to your home to assist you at self-birthing, contact the American College of Home Obstetrics, 664 North Michigan Avenue, Suite 600, Chicago, Illinois 60611.

Specific Home Birth Classes by ACHI

From one small group in Arlington, Massachusetts, founded in October 1972 by lay midwife Tonya Brooks, the Association for Childbirth at Home, International (ACHI), has grown to worldwide proportions. ACHI offers a variety of services, including the only instructional series of classes for laypersons to learn how to birth their own children at home without outside assistance. However, most couples choose to have supervising midwives or physicians, if they are available.

The ACHI educational series is founded on the understanding that giving birth is a joyful and creative act of life in which mother and father can take responsibility for childbirth. With the necessary information provided them, parents plan their own birthing experience, choose the environment in which it will be held, and make ready for any emergency. These formal classes are just about the only place parents can go for basic obstetrical data to prepare them thoroughly for home birth. Classes are given by regionally placed home birth teachers who have gone through ACHI training courses and become certified.

In six sessions that cost a variable amount in different parts of the country but seem to average about $60 per session per couple, instruction is given on the following topics:

- Session 1: *The Advantages of Home Birth*, including the pros and cons of home and hospital birth; the prerequisites for home birth, contraindications to home birth, patients' rights.
- Session 2: *The Normal Birth*, including labor and delivery— what to expect, equipment and supplies, the home birth team, your emergency backup plan.
- Session 3: *The Psychological Issues*, including nonviolent birth for baby and mother, approaching labor and birth, dealing with fear, birth and the family, your sexuality.
- Session 4: *The Medical Considerations*, including high-risk factors discovered in prenatal care, difficulties which may arise in

labor or delivery and what needs to be done, if you need a hospital.

- Session 5: *The Preparations for Birth*, including breathing tools for labor and delivery, exercises, massage techniques.
- Session 6: *The Newborn*, including its nursing, the newborn examination, a check sheet for parents, the neonatal and postpartum period.

To acquire information relating to formal home birth classes held near you, contact the Association for Childbirth at Home, International, Box 1219, Cerritos, California 90701. Telephone: (714) 994-5880.

Informed Homebirth Taped Cassettes

As a defector from ACHI, Rahima Baldwin founded Informed Homebirth, Inc., in Boulder, Colorado. Informed Homebirth is a nonprofit educational organization dedicated to providing pregnant couples with information about birth and the alternatives that are available to them. The participants make their own decisions about the nature and quality of their birth experience.

To reclaim the right to *give* birth, Mrs. Baldwin writes in her manual for parents, *Informed Homebirth*: "We must understand normal birth and the complications which can arise, and prepare ourselves physiologically, psychologically and mentally. We feel that when the parents want a homebirth, when they are well-prepared, and when there are no risk factors jeopardizing safety, the birth will be both safer and more joyful if carried out within the home environment."

Homebirth classes are given by Informed Homebirth, Inc. Because it is a new and regional group, the organization distributes cassette tapes designed to be used in close conjunction with workbooks in a program of self-study. The twelve taped lessons, supplemented by six workbooks, at a cost of $49.75, cover the following subjects:

1. *Why Homebirth?* The advantages of homebirth. Is it safe?
2. *Can I Have My Baby at Home?* Prenatal care. Risk factors that can be found through prenatal screening. Prerequisites for a safe homebirth.
3. *Finding a Skilled Birth Attendant.* Securing emergency backup. Supplies for homebirth.
4. *Normal Labor and Delivery.* Anatomy and physiology. First, second, and third stages. What is it like from the mother's and the birth attendant's points of view?

5. *Relaxation, Breathing and Pushing.* Relaxation is the key to labor. The Kitzinger techniques. Pushing is different at home! "Breathing the baby out."
6. *Relaxation, Breathing and Pushing.* Exercises to practice daily.
7. *Complications and Emergencies, Part I.* Those predictable in advance. Those that can occur during labor and delivery.
8. *Complications and Emergencies, Part II.* Those of the third stage. The newborn in distress. Options if you have to go to the hospital.
9. *The Homebirth Team.* Normal birth from the point of view of the mother, coach, and birth attendant. Taped sequence of an actual birth.
10. *Spiritual and Psychological Aspects.* The Leboyer techniques. Whom to invite. Sexuality and body image.
11. *The Newborn.* Immediate care of the baby. Newborn examination. Other considerations.
12. *The Post-Partum Period.* The mother's health and nutrition. Sexuality. Family adjustment. Getting support. Breast feeding.

Informed Homebirth, Inc., offers membership for $10 and a tape-rental plan at $10 installments. You can receive more information if you write to Carole Tryjanowski, Manager, Informed Homebirth, Inc., P.O. Box 788, Boulder, Colorado 80302. Telephone: (303) 494-0866.

Other Major Home Birth Informational Sources

The National Association of Parents and Professionals for Safe Alternatives in Childbirth (NAPSAC), started by Lee Stewart, C.C.E., and her husband, David Stewart, Ph.D., is dedicated to examining and establishing family-centered childbirth programs that provide the safe aspects of medical science. Toward this end, NAPSAC holds an annual conference during the month of May. The association is striving to attain an ideal—hospitals working in harmony with birth centers which in turn work in harmony with home birth programs. NAPSAC says that parents must not be forced to choose one option to the exclusion of another but should be able to remain flexible, shifting from one facility to another, as developing circumstances indicate, and with a continuity of personnel. To provide information for parents-to-be that will enable them to assume more personal responsibility for pregnancy, childbirth, infant care, and child rearing, NAPSAC publishes pamphlets and books and engages in research projects. The NAPSAC Institute for Childbirth and Family Research is implementing a pilot program to incorporate and refine its ideals.

For more information about its various programs and conferences, contact the National Association of Parents and Professionals for Safe Alternatives in Childbirth, P.O. Box 1307, Chapel Hill, North Carolina 27514. Telephone: (919) 732-7302.

The Society for the Protection of the Unborn through Nutrition (SPUN), was organized by Tom Brewer, M.D. It has been established to reduce the incidence of underweight and premature babies, and concomitantly, the rates of mental retardation, cerebral palsy, hyperactivity, and other disorders. SPUN counsels pregnant women on the fundamentals of prenatal nutrition. It provides speakers for health care meetings, classes, and community groups, produces films, and publishes a semimonthly newsletter and pamphlets.

For more information about how you can benefit from these activities, contact the Society for the Protection of the Unborn through Nutrition, 17 North Wabash, Suite 603, Chicago, Illinois 60602. Telephone: (312) 332-2334. For the Toxemia Hot-Line of SPUN, telephone (914) 271-6471.

To acquire almost any book in print relating to childbirth such as books on midwifery, obstetrics, parenting, home birth, and other alternative birth choices, contact the Childbirth Education Supply Center, 10 Sol Drive, Carmel, New York 10512. Telephone: (914) 225-7763. Or contact the ACHI Bookstore, P.O. Box 1219, Cerritos, California 90701. Telephone: (213) 802-1020. You can receive a current book list at no charge from either book center.

Another place for books and literature is the International Childbirth Education Association (ICEA or CEA). We have described the ICEA previously in Chapter 1. Its slogan is "Freedom of Choice Through Knowledge of Alternatives." What we had not mentioned is that ICEA has a supply center that puts out free current book lists, sells basic childbirth books, and affords information about pediatric care, aspects of parenting, father participation, instructor training, and other items of interest. To receive newsletters, journals, directories, news of regional events—all relating to childbirth—contact the ICEA Supplies Center, P.O. Box 70258, Seattle, Washington 98107.

The Various Items Needed for Home Delivery

What are the various items to have on hand for a home delivery? Our intent is not to give guidelines for labor and obstetrical techniques. Those may be learned from the information sources supplied above or in the appendices. However, if couples are destined to become parents in their own homes, we want to offer the proper tools and instruments with which to deliver the newborn expeditiously.

In order to provide accurate information, we went to two couples who at the time were certified trainers in the educational series for laypersons offered by the Association for Childbirth at Home, International. John and Sue Crockett of Carmel, New York, and Sharon and Richard Roth of Ridgefield, Connecticut, sat for our interviews, showed us films of home births, introduced us to couples who told of their home birth experiences, and provided us with the information presented below. John Crockett has since become certified with Informed Homebirth, Inc., and dropped his affiliation with ACHI. And Sue Crockett has moved to Cerritos, California, to run the ACHI Bookstore. The supplies for home obstetrics you will want to have on hand are the following:

An important piece of equipment is a *rubber syringe* with which to aspirate the baby. While most home-born babies breathe spontaneously, a syringe must be available in case yours does not.

You need a couple of *large bowls* or baby bathtubs for catching the afterbirth; or a tub might be suitable as a temporary crib. Its other logical use, of course, is to carry through with the gentle delivery techniques recommended by Dr. Leboyer—to bathe the newborn. The Roths suggest that a deep Styrofoam cooler works better for the Leboyer bath, since it is deeper and helps to maintain the water temperature. The Crocketts, on the other hand, do not encourage the use of the Leboyer bath at all. They prefer that the newborn's protective film, the *vernix caseosa*, stay on the skin as long as possible.

Additional miscellaneous items are needed such as a *blunt-nose scissors*—best for cutting the cord. It is good, too, to have *boiling water* ready for sterilizing things, and rubbing alcohol. Really important are two pairs of six-inch, curved *Kelly clamps* (hemostat-like instruments for holding the cord), *soap*, and *sterile gloves*. Make sure baby clothes are presoftened by washing. Store cotton swabs, sanitary napkins, receiving blankets, and diapers. *Dental floss* makes a useful string for tying off the umbilical cord, but baby shoelaces are better.

The ACHI instructors said that at birth the room temperature should be at least 75 degrees Fahrenheit. Keep the noise level low, since the infant does better in quiet. Dim the lights, since brightness in the baby's eyes will prevent his or her eye contact with the mother. Upon putting the child on the mother's abdomen, place a warmed receiving blanket over them; that will allow skin-to-skin contact without the exposed surfaces getting chilled. Have a person present who is skilled in cardiopulmonary resuscitation (CPR), in case of need.

Altogether, the Crocketts and the Roths listed thirty-four separate items recommended for birthing at home. The use of each one is explained in the ACHI home birth classes. The reason for following certain obstetrical procedures are also given.

Some home birth groups, including the ACHI, now sell prepackaged equipment kits for birthing at home, such as plastic sheets, bed pads, alcohol, gauze pads, syringes, and cord clamps. And home birth services have been formalized into a business in several cities. For example, the Maternity Center Associates, Ltd. in Bethesda, Maryland, offers a home birth service staffed by nurse-midwives. Sometimes the presence of a skilled birth attendant is necessary; certainly she offers peace of mind to the prospective parents when and if needed. To be safe, be sure to have a well-planned emergency backup system, including preregistration at the local hospital.

The Competency You Should Look for in Home Birth Attendants

The vice-president of the American College of Home Obstetrics, Mayer Eisenstein, M.D., declared in a lecture to NAPSAC that the home birth medical attendant must bring two attributes into play. One is a philosophical attitude which says: "Nature was very wise when she devised this system of reproduction over the thousands and thousands of years. This is a philosophy that will exclude many medical attendants from attending home birth."

The second attribute Dr. Eisenstein spoke of was technical skills. He said, "The medical attendant must bring skills to be able to evaluate labor. The only way you obtain this is by training with someone who is very skillful. This person must realize when labor is normal and when it is abnormal. It sounds like such a simple differentiation, but it is the major one. It is the major thing to know that there is something wrong and decide that, 'I need help,' or 'I can handle it myself.' The medical attendant must be skilled in the diagnosis of problems . . . and in the resuscitation of the newborn."[2]

Other than that, the medical attendant should stand aside, the obstetrician said, so that the mother can deliver herself with the assistance of her husband. "The medical attendant is the guardian of the birth. He or she is the lifeguard. . . . Ninety-five percent of all births are normal, and in those cases it is the role of the medical attendant not to interfere."[3]

From our interviews with couples who have birthed their own babies, we have learned that almost all who have planned for the event in advance did desire a home birth attendant. But often none could be found and, therefore, the birth may have gone unattended. The woman birthed herself with her mate's assistance.

"Our stand is firmly that the ideal situation is a home birth attended by a qualified obstetrical professional," said Sharon Roth, the ACHI instructor, "and we encourage parents to try their hardest to find one. However, there are many home births attended by no doctor and/or midwife, for the simple fact that there are none available in most areas. We have great difficulty in even obtaining prenatal care. And in the end, the responsibility for the pregnancy, birth, and its outcome belongs to the parents."

The Dangers of Childbirth at Home

Although she is a strong proponent of family-centered birth, Delphine Jewell, a certified nurse-midwife who is teaching at the University of Tulsa, is "frightened no end" by the growing trend toward home deliveries. Additionally, she is an outspoken opponent of "lay midwifery" and the dangers that attend such births.

Delphine Jewell's opinions are typical of the kind of opposition put forth by the medical establishment against childbirth at home. It ranges from the benign but unhelpful attitude on the part of most doctors who simply will not consider being present at home births, to the more serious stance of those who refuse prenatal care to women planning home births. Some hospitals have been known to refuse emergency assistance to women who wanted to deliver at home but developed serious complications.

Those complications are what the American College of Obstetricians and Gynecologists (ACOG) were conscious of when it stated its position on "Out-of-Hospital Maternity Care" in January 1976. Its position paper says:

> Labor and delivery, while a physiologic process, clearly presents potential hazards to both mother and fetus, before and after birth. These hazards require standards of safety which are provided in the hospital setting and cannot be matched in the home situation.
>
> We recognize, however, the legitimacy of the concern of many that the events surrounding birth be an emotionally satisfying experience for the family. The College supports those actions that improve the experience of the family while continuing to provide the mother and her infant with accepted standards of safety available only in the hospital.

The officers and directors of ACOG, who are themselves physicians, believe there is insufficient data about the safety of home birth. They are fearful of certain dangers inherent in childbirth in general, and are mindful that any complication happening in the hospitals can certainly happen at home.

One of the complications of childbirth is the condition of *breech birth,* which is the presentation of a fetus where its buttocks are closest to the cervix in one of three postures: the complete breech, the frank breech, or the footling breech. In the illustrations depicted here, we are looking at the new mother with her pelvic bones upright. She is in a semi-sitting position.

Beginning with Figure 36, we see the *complete breech* where the baby is sitting in the womb with its legs crossed.

Figure 37 shows the baby boy in a position of *frank breech* where he is sitting with both legs straightened up alongside his body and face.

Figure 38 depicts the *footling breech* in which the fetus has one or both of its feet lying below the buttocks.

In all three postures of breech birth, the baby's buttocks are nearer the cervix rather than its head. This is an abnormal position and complicates the process of giving birth to the child.

Another danger is the disproportionately sized fetus, which is a condition whereupon the fetal head does not fit well into, down, or through the mother's pelvis. The baby can be too big for the outlet (cephalopelvic) and get stuck half in and half out.

A third danger is hemorrhaging of the mother from *placenta previa*, where the placenta comes out before the baby, causing the loss of large quantities of blood. The placenta is a highly vascular organ and is attached to the maternal uterine wall. We are aware of one woman who did have this type of hemorrhaging. She got most of the placenta out but left a piece of it inside and had to seek professional help fast. She arrived at the hospital emergency room almost dead from loss of blood. The woman and her husband figured they could control the condition themselves, but they were wrong. The baby was born dead!

A further danger is *prolonged labor*, where the mother is fully dilated and ready to deliver the baby, but the baby refuses to come out. Prolonged labor is a less urgent problem, and the baby will be birthed eventually, but the woman grows weaker and more tired while she waits. She chooses to remain in discomfort for an excessively long time when she could be helped with suitable medication.

A serious complication is *toxemia*, also known as *preeclampsia*. Preeclampsia that is severe enough so that convulsions and even coma occur is called *eclampsia*. Eclampsia can be prevented to a great extent by vigilant prenatal care and competent management of preeclampsia.

Then there is distress of the baby during labor that may not be

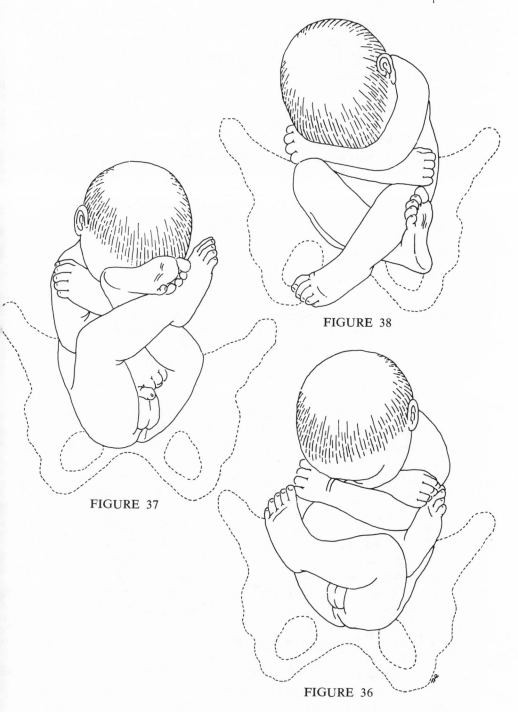

FIGURE 38

FIGURE 37

FIGURE 36

detectable if no one is there to listen to the baby with a stethoscope or has the skill to recognize fetal distress when it is occurring. For instance, if the baby's cord is being compressed by its head, no more than five minutes can elapse with the total shutting off of oxygen or the baby will be dead.

The medical establishment represented by ACOG points out that birth is not 100 percent without risk under any circumstances, either in or out of the hospital. There will always be an irreducible minimum of complications resulting in disability and death during childbirth no matter what measures are taken. Consequently, ACOG has taken a position that though technology may be used to excess in the hospital, it can save lives when applied to the 5 percent of births that are not normal.

The Benefits of Birthing at Home

The people with whom we spoke who are pro-home birth do not deny that there are dangers involved with the procedure. The possible risks are real, they say, but not likely. Hospital births pose certain problems and risks, too, as does riding in a vehicle in city traffic. In the end, they declare the benefits of home birth are well worth the risks. Advocates have shown that the benefits of birthing at home are the following:

Parents control how the mother is treated and avoid unnatural restraints such as delivery table stirrups. The husband can support his wife, nursing the newborn is carried out at once, no pubic shave or enema or episiotomy is performed on the mother, no drugs or anesthetics are given that may affect the baby. "The great thing at home," says Cyril Press, M.D., a surgeon whose wife gave birth to their fourth child at home, "is the absence of harassment. In the hospital there's always a nurse who thinks she knows better than the mother."[4]

Loving friends and relatives can be present. The birthing can be treated as a special event which it is. There can be a glowing fire in the fireplace, soft music playing on the phonograph, the scent of fresh flowers, a bucket of ice chips handy, complete privacy—whatever the couple wants. The couple is surrounded by people they trust who cheer them on.

Labor seems to come to a conclusion faster when the mother is relaxed at home.[5] Perhaps the labor only appears shorter because a woman continues to do routine jobs around the house. She can walk where she wants; take light nourishment such as tea and honey, juices, or yogurt; attend to her own body with a shower or other preparations. So many things can be done to oneself when there are no restraints applied that would go against hospital policy. For example, nothing of a nourishing nature may be eaten in the hospital in case general anesthesia would be needed and the individual could then vomit and choke. Toomis Sauks, M.D., who practices family medicine in Toronto, agrees that labor does progress faster when a woman is relaxed in her own home.[6]

Siblings are not neglected. Other children in the family become part of the big event, they are talked to and played with, their lunches are made for taking to school, no mad dash to the hospital leaves them behind to be cared for by others for a lengthly period. This nonneglect causes siblings to be more accepting of the new little stranger in their midst. The baby becomes their special present.

The father becomes intimately involved with his newborn immediately.[7] Phyllis Curry, C.N.M., said, "The father is involved in a much more meaningful way at home; he's a vital support, not a germ-laden intruder."[8] In a study, the Childbirth Research Institute compared three different types of birth—anesthetized, natural childbirth in the hospital, and home delivery—and found that birthing at home caused nurturing behavior in fathers. There was more parental-infant bonding.

Immediate and firm parental-infant attachment takes place at home. No one removes the child for weighing, labeling, and footprinting. Breast feeding is given at once, and often thereafter. The mother experiences her newborn with all her senses; the natural mother instinct is satisfied by her touching, smelling, and looking at the baby. Mutual imprinting takes place from constant eye-to-eye contact (see Chapter 21).[9]

The medical expense is minimal compared to costs for hospital care given by highly skilled obstetrical specialists. Since pregnancy is an elective event, health insurance policies do not reimburse for hospital and physician attention to childbirth to the same extent as they do for unanticipated medical problems. Insurance companies point out that childbirth is not a disease but a perfectly normal state that can be accomplished by unskilled persons in most instances. Payment is little or none at all with some policies.

However, Informed Homebirth educator John Crockett told us that the cheap cost of home birth should not be a factor. Crockett said, "The least important benefit of home birth is financial. I get scared when a couple sends me vibrations that they are staying home for the monetary savings. I read the riot act to them. I explain that they are only going to save about one thousand dollars. 'Is your spare time worth five dollars an hour?' I ask. 'Then you should spend about two hundred hours preparing for this home birth.' I know that if they spend half that time studying and preparing, they will become quite skilled at taking responsibility for learning about birthing themselves. They must do advance planning and make preparations for home birth; without that the couple is inviting disaster."

The Gentle Home Birth of Stephen Mascia

After six years of marriage Susanne and James Mascia had a baby at home in Wallingford, Connecticut. "Ever since I was a little girl I have dreamed that when I was going to have a baby my husband and I would stay together at home, and then he, our baby, and I would go back to bed together," said Sue Mascia.

"I always thought it was the natural thing to do," Jim Mascia said. "Both of my parents and ten uncles and aunts on my mother's side were all born at home. We knew it wasn't in vogue just now, but it was something we wanted to do for the benefits that come from birthing at home. So Sue prepared herself with a lot of studying."

"I read baby books and articles for three years before I became pregnant. I talked with any authority I could find including nurses, doctors, home birth couples, and women in groups." Mrs. Mascia keeps a bookshelf filled with the latest books on childbirth in her living room.

"Sue received prenatal care at Yale-New Haven Hospital," said Jim. "The midwives examined her on a regular schedule and never found anything wrong. We definitely believed then and still believe that birthing is safer at home. We have heard loads of horror stories from our friends of what they went through in the hospital during labor. There is too much interference by doctors who want to try out their technology."

"Besides, I trust Jim implicitly. I knew he would help me in every way; he studied, and I studied, and at the dinner table every evening we shared our knowledge. Our nutrition is excellent, anyway," Sue said. (Jim Mascia is president of the New England Natural Food and Farming Association, Inc.) "The nurse-midwives at Yale-New Haven couldn't understand why I didn't have any kind of discomfort throughout my pregnancy. 'Are you sure?' they'd ask. 'Don't you get headaches, morning sickness, constipation, back pain?' They kept giving me prescriptions for drugs I never needed or took. Jim and I ate well-balanced meals from fresh, unprocessed foods and took generous amounts of natural vitamin and mineral supplements. We would also ride ten-speed bicycles and walk two miles daily. In fact, both of us do this all the time including throughout my pregnancy right up to the last day."

"We did make arrangements with our friend, a lay midwife in Hartford, who agreed to drive the half hour to our home and attend Sue during the delivery. We understood that I would participate, cut the cord, and do things like that, but Sue was actually going to birth her own baby, while I was to catch it."

"It was a Thursday morning after we had attended a symposium on good nutrition at the Wethersfield High School auditorium that I felt a few labor contractions. At about six A.M. I woke Jim to time the contractions while we lingered in bed until seven o'clock. We got up and had breakfast. I washed dishes, made the bed, sterilized sheets, did a little housecleaning, made ready the various items for birthing, spoke with friends on the phone, wrote letters, and waited. Jim had to go to his office nearby, that morning. After he left, my contractions were five minutes apart, but irregular. I walked through them, breathing as I had been taught in prepared childbirth classes."

"She telephoned our lay midwife," said Jim, "who suggested that she go for an examination at Yale-New Haven Hospital to determine if this was true or false labor, because her contractions were not coming steadily. They sometimes stopped for fifteen minutes."

"I decided to call my nurse-midwife, who had been seeing me at the clinic for prenatal care. Jim came home and drove me to the hospital. It was five thirty P.M. and the clinic was closed. I had to go into the main hospital building alone because parking is impossible in New Haven. After waiting an hour I was examined and learned that I was going to have my baby very soon. The nurses wanted to admit me to the hospital, but I refused and drove back home as fast as possible."

"We were home within a half hour," said Jim, "and I called the lay midwife, our parents, friends, and other relatives. Susanne kept breathing the proper way and walked through her frequent contractions. They were strong and almost doubled her over. She felt she did not want to lie down or sit. I put on our favorite stereo music, made a gallon of herb tea, and put out cookies and other natural food snacks that Sue had made ahead of time for the people who were coming. Then the lay midwife arrived with two other midwives and an M.D. in psychiatry from the University of Connecticut Health Center, who was married to one of the lay midwives. We agreed that he could watch our reactions to birthing ourselves. His intent was to write a clinical journal article about his observations."

"I had various little 'nests' ready for myself," said Sue; "they included the bed, lots of pillows piled on the floor, a little stool, and an old easy chair, because I didn't know where I was going to want to be. I labored in all of them, trying each in turn. The stool was too low to the ground. The easy chair was too soft—insufficient leverage from which to push. I laid on the pillows. I laid on my back in bed. Then the midwives examined me and found I was fully dilated. It was time to make up my mind. I decided to deliver on my hands and knees on the bed. On all fours seemed like the most comfortable and natural position for me. They put disposable diapers under me, and I worked through a few contractions that way. Since I couldn't stand any kind of clothing on me, I was completely naked. Jim was right there along with everyone else."

"We were all doing something to help," said the father. "I gave her ice chips and whispered encouraging words in her ear. The psychiatrist took pictures of the whole thing and tape-recorded all the sounds. One midwife massaged Sue's perineum with wheat germ oil so that she opened more and was lubricated. Her contractions were coming hard and frequently, and then the bag of waters broke all over me. In a little while I saw our baby's head crowning. It wasn't a blond."

"Baby Stephen came out with no problem. I hardly pushed at all, and no episiotomy was needed even with this being my first baby. I had no tearing or stretch marks. He just slid out nice and easy and very fast. The lights were low, we spoke softly, did everything slow and relaxed, and Jim or the midwife were ready to catch the baby. Actually, baby Stephen began crying while his shoulders, hips, and legs were still inside of me."

"It was amazing!" said James Mascia about his son. "Only his head was protruding into the world when he began crying. Then his shoulders came along with the rest of him. He turned pink immediately. His eyes were already open as he appeared, and he seemed to be looking all around the room. The child was remarkably clean—no cheesy covering like you see in some movies of newborns. There were no blobs of blood or other ugly marks on him either. He looked to be a healthy little boy that might be four or five days old."

"Baby Stephen did get blood on him when he waited near my back end still attached by his umbilical cord. The midwives had to draw blood into a test tube for the Rh negative test. Yes, I am Rh negative, which did not stop me from having a home birth. Our New Haven pediatrician, Dr. Morris Wessel, kept close tabs on what we were doing. For instance, he interviewed us months before to assure himself that we were responsible people, and he gave us the test tube to bring in the blood for testing. Jim, Stephen, and I visited Dr. Wessel that same birthing day for Stephen's examination. The doctor took blood specimens from both of us for further laboratory examination. The baby and I were just fine. Like me, Stephen was born Rh negative so that I needed no special gamma globulin injection—'Rho Gam'—to make my next pregnancy safe. The pediatrician immediately took our blood samples to the laboratory himself."

"After her midwife took the blood sample directly following my

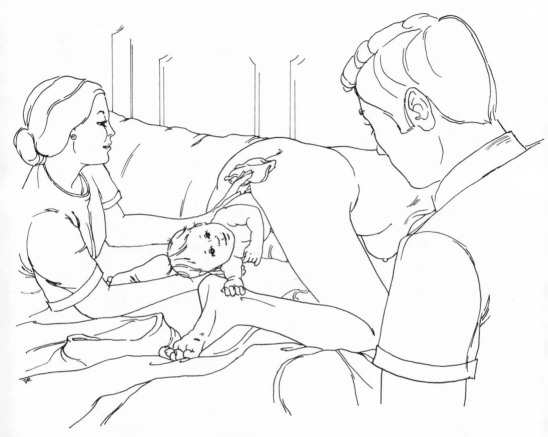

FIGURE 39

son's birth, I tied the umbilical cord with an aseptic shoelace," said
Jim Mascia. "Then the midwife cut the cord and handed Stephen to
Sue. She held him to her breast for suckling. In about twenty minutes
she felt the afterbirth starting to come and therefore handed the baby
back to to me. My shirt was off so I held him against my bare chest for
skin-to-skin contact, and we gazed into each other's eyes."

"The midwives left about two thirty A.M. Jim buried the placenta in
our garden between the tomato plants. We cleaned up the rooms,
talked awhile, and went to bed with the baby lying between us as we
held hands. It was what I had always pictured. We slept a little, then
arose, raring to go. I felt I just had to get out and show people my
baby. He was so beautiful!" said the new mother.

"Before visiting the pediatrician that afternoon, we went to the
Wallingford town hall to record Stephen's birth, but the town clerk
did not know how to fill out a birth certificate. She was the Walling-

ford town clerk for seventeen years and never had been called upon to do it in all that time," said Jim. "In fact, it was difficult even to convince the town hall officials that our baby had been born at home just a few hours earlier."

That evening, the proud parents took baby Stephen to visit his grandparents. All of them dined together and celebrated.

The next day, the new family went grocery shopping. All three of them were out and around visiting friends throughout most of Saturday.

After he had attended church with his parents, we saw baby Stephen Mascia on Sunday, less than three days following his birth. He appeared alert, pink, smiling, and intrigued with his surroundings. The little boy looked as though he already were at least two weeks old. His pretty mother seemed in wonderful condition, too.

Jim Mascia presided with his family present at a well-attended meeting of the Connecticut chapter of the Natural Food and Farming Association. The guest speaker's topic was "holistic health," and as he spoke baby Stephen smacked his lips while snacking at his mother's breast.

NOTES FOR CHAPTER NINETEEN

1. Gregory White and Mayer Eisenstein, "The American College of Home Obstetrics (ACHO) Philosophy and Practice of Physicians in Home-birth," *21st Century Obstetrics Now!* ed. Lee Stewart and David Stewart (Chapel Hill, N.C.: The National Association of Parents and Professionals for Safe Alternatives in Childbirth, 1977).

2. White and Eisenstein, "ACHO Philosophy."

3. White and Eisenstein, "ACHO Philosophy."

4. Fredelle Maynard, "Home Births vs. Hospital Births," *Woman's Day,* June 28, 1977.

5. N. Newton, D. Peeler, and M. Newton, "Effects of Disturbance on Labor," *American Journal of Obstetrics and Gynecology* 101:1096 (1968).

6. Maynard, "Home Births."

7. Newton et al., "Effects of Disturbance."

8. Maynard, "Home Births."

9. Marshall H. Klaus and John H. Kennell, *Maternal-Infant Bonding* (St. Louis: C.V. Mosby Co., 1976).

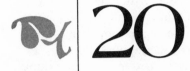

20

When the Baby Arrives: The Breast Is Best

Babies who have trouble learning to eat are usually the ones who have not been offered their mothers' breasts soon after birth. The nursing instinct is very strong as soon as the baby has his breathing well enough coordinated so that he can suck and swallow and breathe. With most babies that is immediately after birth; with those who have mucus or are drugged, it takes longer; but like many other learning patterns in children, if the sucking desire is thwarted when it first arises, the baby gets discouraged and may have to be taught to suck later.
—LESTER DESSEZ HAZELL, M.D.,
Commonsense Childbirth

The Age of the Bosom

Advertising, movies, books, fashions, and television have glamorized the breast and distorted its natural function. It is now linked with sex rather than with its primary purpose, to give milk to the newborn. We live in the age of the bosom.

Adding to this focus on bust lines as sex symbols, improved methods and facilities have made formula feeding simple and safe. It is much more convenient for the doctor to suggest a formula. He or she can easily prescribe a proper amount of mineral and iron requirements and figure out the correct caloric content in a formula. What you shouldn't overlook, however, is that no formula—no matter how nutritious or perfectly balanced—has been able to duplicate mother's milk. To this day chemists have been baffled in their efforts to analyze all of the ingredients. They have been able to develop some good imitations of mother's milk—but as yet, no exact duplication.

For feeding your baby, the breast is best, in our opinion. Many doctors feel that it is so important for a woman to breast-feed that every effort should be made to do so even if only for a short time. The greatest gift that you can give your child is part of yourself, the milk of your body. Breast feeding unites the two of you in a bond of love and good health.

Breast feeding aids in restoring your figure more quickly to its normal, nonpregnant state. As the baby sucks on your nipples, it stimulates contractions of the uterus, which help expel remaining bits of lining tissue inside the uterus. Thus, the nursing mother's uterus returns to its normal size faster than does the nonnursing mother's. Breasts being stimulated by an infant's sucking also produce natural oxytocin to contract the uterus and reduce the risk of postpartum bleeding.

Breast feeding temporarily eliminates, delays, or reduces the menstrual flow and preserves your iron reserve. Giving milk is enjoyable, sexually arousing, and restful, and a wonderful feeling of satisfaction comes over you as you watch your child take in nourishment. Finally, by your breast feeding, naturally functioning glands don't go haywire and there may be less risk of getting breast cancer.

Baby cries less often because his or her physical need is satisfied so quickly by breast milk. The process is cheaper, easier, safer, and faster than feeding with refrigerated formula or sterilized bottles. Breast milk has all the necessary food elements baby needs, which makes it quickly and easily digested. It's always fresh, stays sterile, and your baby will experience softer stools and less constipation or diarrhea.

A breast-fed baby suffers less from colic, stomach upset, colds, ear infections, and there are fewer skin and facial disorders. Eating problems and dental difficulties will be much reduced or eliminated. Moreover, the baby's feeling of safety and security is assured. A more stable personality is molded by breast feeding. Psychiatrists are of the opinion that the way an adult adapts and adjusts to the world depends on the way his or her basic needs were satisfied from birth. For the sake of completeness we must mention that the baby is also able to sense the attitude of a mother who finds it sickening to feed her infant from the breast.

Specific Medical Benefits from Breast Feeding Baby

Aside from these more general advantages for breast feeding your newborn, there are specific medical benefits the baby will enjoy. They are the following:

- Mother's milk contains antibodies, cells, enzymes, and other factors for the baby's *resistance to environmental irritants.*[1]
- Necessary *iron becomes more readily available* and usable.
- Better appetite control develops.[2]
- *A milk protein* (lactoferrin), *a growth factor* (Lactobacillus bifidus), and *an antistaphylococcal* factor are provided in mother's milk that are not present in man-made formula or in cow's milk.[3]
- Human milk offers baby *longer immunity against diseases,* even outlasting the nursing period. His or her respiratory and gastrointestinal tracts, an infant's major areas of infection, are well protected by secretory antibodies in mother's milk.[4]
- Breast feeding *reduces the incidence of diarrhea* and helps avoid dehydration from severe salt imbalance in the event diarrhea does develop.[5]
- If a cold strikes the infant, *antibodies in human milk* but absent in other foods prevent the virus from turning into more serious respiratory illnesses.[6]
- Breast feeding *lowers the occurrence of ear infections.*[7] Bottle-fed infants get more ear infections from being fed while lying on their backs, thus letting the milk to flow into the middle ear.[8]
- *Less tooth decay* develops in breast-fed babies.
- Foreign proteins in cow's milk may sensitize the newborn infant and lay the foundations for food allergies in later life.[9,10] Thus, breast milk affords *less chance of developing food allergies.*
- There is a *lower risk of obesity* for nursing babies because they stop feeding when they are full. Overanxious mothers will not be inclined to force more food on them simply because the mothers cannot determine how much milk their babies have taken.

The Chemical Consistency of Human Milk

A pediatric neurochemist, Gerald Gaull, M.D., professor of pediatrics at New York's Mount Sinai Medical School and chief of Human Development and Genetics at the New York Institute for

Basic Research in Mental Retardation, pointed out in an interview that milk is "more species-specific and of more special importance to the development of man than we thought."

In other words, *calves* thrive on *cow's* milk and *babies* thrive on *human* milk. Cow's milk is the usual base for artificial baby formula. Analysis reveals that whey makes up 60 percent of the proteins in human milk, while caseins account for 40 percent. Bovine milk (from the cow) has protein that is 18 percent whey and 82 percent casein. That is too much casein for a human infant to digest.

Dr. Gaull further states that caseins contain little of the sulfur amino acid cystine that babies need; but it contains too much phenylalanine and tyrosine, which are the aromatic amino acids that newborns do not digest well until much later. Mother's milk has just the right amounts of these amino acids, and has a higher percentage of unsaturated fats than does bovine milk. It has the correct quantity of vitamin E to prevent swelling in infants as well.

The pediatric scientist also said that a nonprotein nitrogen compound called *taurine* is two times more abundant in breast milk than in cow's milk. He is amassing "considerable evidence that taurine is of nutritional significance in brain development, and that it may be a neurotransmitter or neuromodulator substance in brain and retina [eyes]."[11]

Our own investigation of the medical literature indicates that breast milk is a far superior form of nutrition for an infant. While many formulas try to simulate breast milk, none as yet has been successful in duplicating this amazing substance. Simply, the protein in breast milk is of a different nature than the protein in formulas, although there is no reason why a breast-fed infant cannot have an occasional bottle. Furthermore, there are tremendous pressures on parents today to introduce solid foods as early as possible. We advise you to resist these pressures. Some infants begin solids at one week; most are on solids by six weeks. In both instances, this is too soon. An infant will grow and develop adequately on breast milk alone for the first four to six months of life. No solid food is needed.

The Resurgent Popularity of Breast Feeding in America

A recent survey by a formula manufacturer indicated that nearly two out of five American mothers now breast-feed their infants. This is double the percentage of fifteen years ago. The advent of the new better-educated, more-prepared parents has created this resurgent popularity of breast feeding in America. Mothers feel a growing pride and emotional satisfaction in nourishing their babies from their own bodies. Convenience and economy are also factors. Today's parents want to give their children what nature provided, don't wish to waste a "natural resource," and realize that breast milk is healthier for their babies.

The American Academy of Pediatrics, in 1976, urged physicians to encourage breast feeding as a means of infant nutrition that "has not been improved on." In March 1977, researchers announced at a New York Academy of Sciences meeting that human milk is superior to formula based on bovine milk because it gives the infant high energy and fatty acids to promote the development of the central nervous system. Bovine milk gives high protein content to increase body size and muscle mass quickly, something calves need but not human infants. Thus, cow's milk may start a child on the path to overnutrition, a tendency toward obesity and large body size that would require a lifetime of high-protein foods.

Smart women today have exposed themselves to this information and are shunning the effects of overnutrition for their infants. They know that in American culture, such eating is high in animal proteins. Cow's milk during infancy may promote a life-style conducive to heart disease, colon and breast cancer, and other degenerative diseases that are on the increase in our society. Bottle feeding of newborns may be a causative factor.

La Leche League International, Inc., will celebrate its silver anniversary in 1981. The La Leche League is made up of informed women and some men who sponsor discussion groups led by certified consultants to help women who want to nurse. There are groups all over the country. A series of four monthly meetings costs $8. Those interested can write to La Leche League International, 9616 Minneapolis Avenue, Franklin Park, Illinois 60134, or telephone (312) 455-7730.

Preparing for Breast Feeding

To get ready for confident, comfortable breast feeding, there are several easy finger exercises that you can practice during the last six to eight weeks of pregnancy. These exercises toughen your nipples and prepare your breasts for feeding. It's a matter of simply hand-milking the breasts, coupled with proper hygienic care.

1. Rub the nipples with a wash cloth.
2. Leave the tops down on the bra.
3. Express milk with gentle squeezing.
4. Pull out on the nipple.
5. Use no soap on the breasts.

Another important way to prepare yourself for breast feeding is to keep in top physical condition and maintain good eating habits with a commonsense diet. You may experience a slight increase in appetite during breast feeding. It is nature's way of signaling you to eat more foods, especially those rich in calcium and protein.

Nursing and Your Sexuality

In what way will breast feeding affect you physically and sexually? What special meaning will it have for you from a woman's viewpoint?

In some women, the hormonal influx stimulated by breast feeding may bring sexual arousal. You might feel more womanly and more interest in your husband. Sometimes a positive birth experience draws you psychologically closer to him, and you feel a greater intimacy than ever before. Breast feeding may heighten this feeling. Small wonder that a husband prefers it to bottle feeding. The bond of sexual love usually is strengthened and deepened by nursing your baby. Of course, some husbands may possibly be turned off by a woman's breast feeding.

But this same hormonal influx affects other perfectly normal women in such a way that they are less interested in sexual intercourse, even though they may feel closer to their mates. Many women who experience a lessening of sexual feelings find that their interest does return slowly and gradually over the months, even as nursing continues.

Heightened sexuality may cause some leakage of milk, which is normal. Hormones released at the time of a woman's climax may cause some of this leakage.

We should advise that no matter what method you choose to feed your baby, interest in sex may be changed after the birth for both mother and father. Sometimes it takes the couple awhile to adjust to their new roles of mother and father. Tensions due to added responsibilities often set in, as well as physical and emotional exhaustion. What is needed is open communication, patience, and acceptance. Any diminished sexual desire is temporary and is in no way abnormal.

Menstruation may be delayed by the feedings but don't be fooled into thinking they are a substitute for birth control. It is not! Use some form of contraception *other than oral contraception* before the return of the first period. The oral contraceptives you took prior to pregnancy should be avoided now because they alter the composition of breast milk. The pills' synthetic hormones will pass into the milk to upset the normal sexual development of the infant. We suggest that you ask your doctor for an alternative form of birth control.

What Is Required for Successful Breast Feeding?

To acquire detailed information about how to achieve successful breast feeding, we consulted with Betsy Hoffman, a certified La Leche League leader in Stamford, Connecticut. Mrs. Hoffman suggested that successful nursing is dependent on three factors: a motivated, well-informed mother; a cooperative, strong-sucking infant; and a physician who encourages it. Mrs. Hoffman said, "Most women, with very few exceptions, are physically able to breast-feed successfully. The problems that surround nursing are mostly psychological, from anxiety or fear about one's ability to nurse. Such anxiety in turn impairs that ability.

"There are, however, some justifiable reasons why a woman chooses not to nurse, and she should not feel that she will somehow shortchange her baby if she follows her instincts. She has her own feelings to consider, as well as her husband's. For one, she may need to return to work as quickly as possible. While this may imply that working and breast feeding are incompatible, they aren't! Breast feeding and keeping a job take much planning and sometimes exhausting effort, but it can be done successfully. Yet a woman may find that breast feeding cuts too much into her time and energy," said Mrs. Hoffman.

The La Leche League leader offered women some additional tips for successful breast feeding:

1. Generally, no matter how small your breasts, almost all mothers will have enough milk. Breast size has nothing to do with milk supply or the number of milk ducts and glands. The size is due to fatty tissue quantity. The breasts often look larger during the time you are nursing, but they will probably return to their original size after the baby is weaned.
2. Nursing consumes from 500 to 1500 calories of energy, depending on your body size, so that you need to eat that much extra food. These calories should come from protein: low-fat milk products, lean meat, fish, and lots of vegetables and fruit. You won't gain weight from eating well-balanced, satisfying meals. Mrs. Hoffman, who was herself a nursing mother when we interviewed her, took no extra minerals or other food supplements. She believes that it is important to drink plenty of liquid—about one eight-ounce glass of liquid each time you nurse to ensure adequate milk. During our interview hours, Betsy Hoffman nursed her baby periodically and sipped herb tea steadily. She suggests that you eat no high-calorie, low-nutrition snacks like sweets and potato chips.

3. You don't have to do anything difficult to prepare your breasts for nursing, as we indicated before. A woman with inverted nipples can follow a corrective, self-administered procedure. Unfortunately, some obstetricians do not pay sufficient attention to the would-be mother's breasts and may not notice that the nipples are inverted. In that case, help yourself. Inversion is easy to diagnose: The nipple goes in instead of out when the edges of the nipple are pinched with the thumb and forefinger. If that happens, you would be able to correct the situation by obtaining a pair of Woolrich shields to wear for progressively longer periods of time once or twice each day two to three months before the newborn is expected. These shields, which are available from the La Leche League, exert a steady, gentle pressure on the inverted nipple to draw it out gradually.

4. For normal nipples, rough-toweling, plus some exercises we described which involve rolling the nipple out once or twice a day for about two months before the infant arrives, is the only preparation needed. A pregnant woman should avoid washing her nipples with soap as it robs the nipple of normal body oils that ordinarily keep them from becoming dried or chapped.

5. Breast milk is a thin, usually bluish fluid, and it will not look as heavy and creamy as ordinary cow's milk. Your baby will be getting proper nutrition from your breast if he or she looks healthy, seems relatively satisfied, and is gaining weight—and is supplying you with plenty of wet diapers. Above all, do not worry about your milk supply, since anxiety can cause a reduction in milk flow.

6. The milk "let down" reflex is felt by many women when their milk actually starts flowing. It is colostrum or "first milk," which begins flowing with sucking. Betsy Hoffman says, "The milk let down reflex has been identified as a tingling or tightening sensation within the breast and is felt by many women when the milk is actually ready to flow. Some women who have lots of milk which gushes forth freely do not feel this sensation, or feel it faintly. Every now and again, a pregnant woman may feel a let-down when she hears an infant cry or thinks of her baby; but as her nursing experience continues, such accidents, where she makes milk before her baby needs it, decrease."

What is most important for us to stress is that milk production is dependent on sucking stimulation of the breasts. The longer and more frequently the baby nurses, the more milk the mother will produce. It is that simple. When your baby is put to your breast and starts sucking, the nerve endings stimulate the pituitary to release prolactin, the hormone which stimulates milk production. After the baby has started

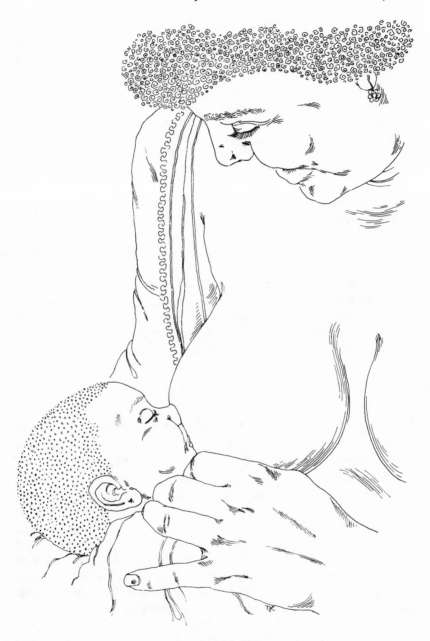

FIGURE 40

sucking is when most mothers feel the let-down. The stronger the sucking, the stronger the feeling of the let down reflex. It is believed by some specialists that weak sucking fails physiologically to trigger the pituitary gland and milk let down is delayed.

7. *Colostrum*, a thick, yellowish substance present in the breasts during the latter part of pregnancy and the first few weeks after birth, is not true milk, but is very important for the newborn. Colostrum is all the baby needs during the first few hours after birth. It has a slightly laxative effect and helps the infant pass the meconium from his bowels. More importantly, it contains every nutrient a newborn needs as well as immunizing factors which will protect his health.

In summary of what we are saying here, the more frequently the mother nurses, the sooner the true milk—that thinner, bluish-white stuff most of us consider breast milk—will come in. Mothers who are not separated from their babies after birth, and who nurse frequently, may have their milk come in less than twenty-four hours. Women who are separated from their babies, because the infants are kept in the nursery, and do not nurse so frequently, may not have their milk for two to four days.

Weaning Your Child Away from Breast Feeding

More often than not, it is societal pressure that dictates when a mother weans her baby away from the breast. Mrs. Hoffman told us that while ages six to nine months are most common in the United States, the time for weaning should come when your child decides to end the breast-feeding relationship and not when peculiar looks come from the neighbors.

If you decide to terminate the breast feeding, weaning should be gradual to avoid any discomfort of overfilled breasts and undue upset to the infant. To do this, replace one breast feeding daily with a bottle feeding. Then a few days later replace another daily feeding with a bottle. If you know that you will be weaning the infant early, transition might be easier if you feed the youngster supplemental bottles occasionally from the first few weeks.

Betsy Hoffman says: "If a mother wants to experience 'baby-led' weaning, she will find that breast milk will completely satisfy her child's nutritional needs for the first half year of its life. A baby will signal the mother that he or she is ready to begin solids, when he starts showing a clear interest in foods at mother's mealtimes; when he has the motor coordination to pick things up and put them into his mouth; and when a mother, after several days of very demanding nursing, finds that no matter how often she nurses and no matter how much her baby drinks, it is simply not enough to satisfy him. That is when you might try some solid food."

Mrs. Hoffman added: "As related to speed feeding, some babies at four or five months can completely empty a breast in five to seven minutes. This does not imply that there is not enough milk; rather, it is more indicative that baby is a very efficient, strong-sucking nurser and that his mom can produce the amount of milk he needs quickly. Moreover, at feeding time a restless, fidgety baby may not be acting that way due to a lack of food; therefore, the mother will have to take a lot into account concerning the weaning process. Too many other factors could be involved in producing restless behavior."

The La Leche League leader recommends that you not use the prepackaged baby foods sold in grocery stores and supermarkets. They have unnecessary sugars and modified starches added to tantalize the palate of the mother, but which has no beneficial effect on the baby. Make your own vegetables, fruits, and meats, mashed soft for easy swallowing, and add them gradually to the milk diet, advises Mrs. Hoffman.

The youngster will take less milk as he or she eats more solid food. In turn, your own breast milk supply will taper off. Less sucking on the breasts reduces milk quantity and discomfort from engorgement should be little or no problem. Complete weaning will be attained when your baby eats solid food and drinks formula or cow's milk without any preference for breast milk.

Any Amount of Nursing Is Important

We emphasize that any amount of nursing is important. Even a small attempt can be a tremendous advantage to both mother and child, as indicated above. Working mothers may feel guilty that they are unable to give time to breast feeding, but they can—at least a little. Breast milk may be expressed manually into bottles and refrigerated for feeding to baby when the mother is not there. In fact, it can be frozen and used even six months later, with the nourishment still sealed in. The technique of manual expression is taught in one of the four educational sessions offered by the La Leche League International, Inc.

There are other psychological and emotional benefits to breast feeding. Nursing stimulates emotional closeness by physical proximity. Your mutual skin contact, eye contact, and your own rocking, cuddling, fondling, and mothering will build a maternal-infant attachment that is vital for your baby's mental health as an adult. In the next chapter we will discuss in more detail this bonding between parents and infant.

Derrick B. Jelliffe, M.D., professor of Public Health and of Pediatrics; head of the Division of Population, Family and International Health, School of Public Health, University of California at Los Angeles, says: "At all ages of life, feeding is much more than the supply of needed nutrients. . . . Recent work suggests increasingly that human milk—or rather, the whole process of breast feeding—has a special significance for both mother and baby, from an emotional and economic point of view. This is in addition to the overwhelming accumulation of scientific data concerning specific nutritional and anti-allergic properties in human milk."

NOTES FOR CHAPTER TWENTY

1. C. Alford et al., "Development Humoral Immunity and Congenital Infections in Man," in *The Immune System and Infectious Diseases*, ed. I. Neter and F. Milgrom (Basel, Switzerland: International Convocation on Immunology, 1975).

2. B. Hall (untitled article), *Lancet* 1:779–81 (1975).

3. A. Goldman and C. Smity, "Host Resistance Factors in Human Milk," *Journal of Pediatrics* 82:1082–1090 (1973).

4. W. Walker and R. Hong, "Immunology of the Gastrointestinal Tract," *Journal of Pediatrics* 83:517–30 (1973).

5. M. Kingston, "Biochemical Disturbance in Bottle Fed Infants with Gastroenteritis and Dehydration," *Journal of Pediatrics* 82:1073–81 (1973).

6. M. Dowham et al. "Breast Feeding Protects Against Respiratory Syncytial Virus Infections," *British Medical Journal* 2:274–76 (1976).

7. T. Wilson, *Diseases of Eye and Ear in Children* (London: William Heineman, 1955).

8. W. Beauregard, "Positional Otitis Media," *Journal of Pediatrics* 79:294–96 (1971).

9. T. Boat et al. "Hyperreactivity to Cow's Milk," *Journal of Pediatrics* 87:23–29 (1975).

10. V. Vaughn and R. McKay, eds., *Nelson Textbook of Pediatrics* (Philadelphia: W. B. Saunders, 1975).

11. Hara Marano, "Infant Development Seen Optimized by Breast Milk," *Medical News*, October 31, 1977.

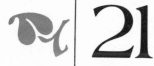 # 21

Parent-Infant Bonding Begins at Birth

They told me babies should not be held;
It would spoil them and make them cry.
I wished to do what is best for them,
And the years went swiftly by,
Now empty are my yearning arms;
No more that thrill sublime.
If I had my babies back again,
I'd hold them all the time.
—A MOTHER *feeling the deepest longing*

What is the culmination of pregnancy that mother and father look for—the bringing forth of a healthy child? No, it is more than that! Good health is desired, of course, but additionally, parents want a bonding—the child attached to the parents and the parents attached to the child.

The complex phenomenon of bonding and attachment is a reciprocal linkage at many levels between the parents and their infant. In definition, an "attachment" is a unique relationship that is particular and endures through time. It includes certain actions of one person to the other involving personal contact and an exhibit of affection. These actions, taken at birth or near to it, will cause an imprinting in the inner recesses of the minds of both parents and child.

This bond begins for the parents even before conception. According to Marshall H. Klaus, M.D., professor of Pediatrics at the Case Western Reserve University School of Medicine and the Rainbow Babies and Children's Hospital, Cleveland, Ohio, bonding is a kind of cellular or chemical process that starts in the mother, and perhaps the father, when they are planning to have a child. Then, when pregnancy is confirmed, the mothering instinct by hormonal or other mechanism builds up steadily to produce a yearning by the woman to fondle her baby. She sees herself doing it. The yearning, deep longing, and mothering instinct are further confirmed by fetal movements inside her, and this reinforces the woman's tender passion even more.

Bonding comes to fruition in the step by step occurrences of giving birth, seeing the child, touching him or her, and rendering care.[1]

What the Ideal Birth Experience May Be

Is there an ideal birth experience that one might look to as an example of parental-infant bonding?

We observed a couple from a rural community having their first baby. It was late at night; she labored in the birthing room of our family-oriented hospital. Her long, sleek hair shone like black satin in the dim light, while the father lingered by her side. Each smiled into the other's brown eyes. There was hardly a sound. They moved together in quiet harmony and grace. He coached her in techniques of breathing, timed the seconds of contractions, slipped ice chips into her mouth, and massaged areas where labor pain caused discomfort.

They were totally relaxed, and the forces of labor were strong. Birthing went quickly while she sat upright in bed holding onto her thighs. The mother had no need even to bear down and merely breathed the baby out. His head bloomed like a rose on the perineum and slid into the attendant's hands. It was simple. Smooth. Nothing said.

She reached down in slow motion and took the child to her breast, quietly and peacefully. Then she cooed whispered words of love as the father stroked the boy's tiny body. His son made sucking noises and pulled at the nipple. The new parents chuckled in satisfaction. Their infant opened his eyes wide to search their faces well, seeming to know them as his parents. He felt safe, nurtured, and supported. Then, some mystical imprint was made and a spiritual energy exchanged, all in silence except for the sounds of the child suckling. The bond was firm—attachment established.

Immediate Bonding Is Related to High Infant Survival Rates

A happy survival in the extrauterine world will most readily be achieved by the infant through attachment bonds with loving parents. This is the case in nature. A characteristic of almost all mammals is the continuous and very close mother-young interaction during the first few minutes and hours of birth. However, while Western man is a mammal, his present culture dictates that he go against mammalian nature by separating the mother from her infant immediately following birth. The result is a profound and probably permanent effect on both the mother and her child.

Separation was not always the practice for mother and newborn; it has been with us only since 1900 when our modern hospital system was instituted. Before that, mothers frequently gave birth at home. Of course, infant deaths then were about 140 out of each 1000 babies born. Today for every 1000 live births infant mortality has decreased to 16.7. Still, fourteen industrial nations have a better live birth record than the United States. In Finland the infant death rate is about 12 per 1000. In Japan it is 11.3, and in Sweden it is under 10. These countries encourage nonseparation of parents and newborn at birth. The better statistics are due to certain factors: social causes with better nutrition and living conditions and parent-infant bonding, the more naturalist approach to childbearing.

Ill-Effects in the Infant of Deprived Parental Bonding

The Scottish psychoanalyst R. D. Laing, M.D., has emerged as a vocal and persuasive champion of maternal-infant bonding. He wrote the script and provided the on- and offscreen commentary for *Birth, with R. D. Laing*, a visually powerful polemic on the inhumanities of childbirth and the treatment of newborn babies as insensate beings. Dr. Laing takes a militant stance as a parent and consumer of medical services and makes an impassioned plea—bolstered by medical data —for sensitive handling of infants and their mothers. He speculates warily on how the birth experience may affect later life and suggests that what happens during childbirth can profoundly influence a baby's life.

"There's a critical period of the first seventy-two hours following birth," Dr. Laing said. "This is just the right time for bonding, when the mother's natural desire is to have her baby and when the baby needs the mother."[2]

Dr. Laing condemned the current hospital procedure of separating the infant from the mother for so-called medical reasons. "Risk of infection is the common excuse," he said, "but the real reason is that it's more convenient for the hospital to keep babies in one central place and mothers in another.

"It's the shattering of these bonds that's a precondition of insanity," he said. "The mother-child interaction is most significant. The disruption of bonding can be one of the causes of schizophrenia in later life." He cites his own findings. "In all radical therapy what patients constantly repeat are gruesome birth experiences. It might be simply a metaphor but the roots of schizophrenia are in catastrophic experiences and birth is one of them. None of us expect to go through in life what we've gone through at birth, outside of torture chambers."[3] This is Dr. Laing's personal opinion from his evaluation of patients. He believes that the birth trauma is an experience all of us carry throughout life.

Besides possible mental illness in adult life, infants who are deprived of bonding within the first few days of birth experience a variety of other problems, including digestive malfunctioning, a sense of abandonment, depression, inability to maintain consistently human relationships, and even dwarfism of deprivation.[4] Yes, Dr. Gardner, in 1972, reported that babies become dwarfed in growth from being deprived of love.

In contrast, cooing and other soft sounds made by parents produce in the baby calm behavior, increased weight gain, early development of perception, recognition, judgment, reasoning, imagination, enhancement of visual tracking, and exploration. In turn, stimulation of these senses in the baby produces an increase in the bonds of attachment.[5,6]

When a developed fetus leaves its warm, nourishing, protected, and familiar uterine environment and enters a new place that is strange, cold, dissatisfying, and possibly life-threatening, the newborn may experience moments of terror, just as the retired French obstetrician Dr. Frederick Leboyer has suggested.

Dr. Laing partially agrees with Dr. Leboyer, "Not only the physical surroundings—which should be warm and comfortable with the technology in the background—but the people and the whole package," Dr. Laing said. "Is the woman the active participant and are other people taking their cues from her? And is the baby being handled the way one would want if he were as helpless as that?"

Dr. Laing speaks out for babies publicly and privately. "I agree with the basic principles of what Leboyer says, although I'm not at all dedicated to the specifics of his method," he said. (See Chapter 15 for the details of Dr. Leboyer's method.) "We should welcome babies with kindness and respect. It's a terrible reflection of our time that a lone voice must speak out on behalf of infants.

"But Leboyer," Dr. Laing added, "is not interested in the mother's insistence that it's her baby. I believe that the mother-baby relationship must be preserved during and after birth."[7]

How might it be preserved to accomplish desirable attachment bonds? What the infant needs at the time of birth is continuation or close approximation of the place from which he or she came, with only a gradual change to something different. Parents can create attachment by using gentle touches, allowing only comforting sights, and furnishing soft sounds. Added to these the strength of the bond and how the infant develops will depend on how much the mother and infant remain together immediately after birth. Our belief, based on our observations and the scientific studies of others, is that they should spend as much time as possible in each other's company during this very sensitive period.[8,9,10]

The "Sensitive Period" in Mothers Following Childbirth

As with the newborn, attachment bonds are formed in the mother during a "sensitive period" following childbirth. This was shown in a 1971 presentation to the American Pediatric Society by Dr. Klaus. In explaining his research findings, Dr. Klaus said, "Major alterations of maternal behavior" will result from permitting the mother of a healthy term infant to have extensive close contact with her infant in the early hours and days of life." He reported his study of twenty-eight primiparous mothers (birthing for the first time) of normal term infants:[11]

Fourteen mothers were changed from the usual hospital procedure of maternal-infant separation. These mothers formed the extended contact group and were allowed to handle their infants for an hour within three hours after birth, and also for fifteen extra hours during the three days following delivery. Another fourteen mothers formed the control group. They had the usual hospital routine: a glimpse of the infant shortly after birth, brief contact and identification at six to twelve hours, and visits of twenty minutes during bottle-feeding every four hours. In 1971, in that particular hospital, breast feeding was considered unusual.

Dr. Klaus undertook his study to determine whether human mothers have a "sensitive period" immediately after delivery, such as has been reported among animal mothers.

In goats, cows, and sheep, separation of the mother and her offspring immediately after birth for a period as short as one hour often results in "unmotherlike" behavior. When the animal infant rejoins the mother, she butts it away or feeds it and other infants indiscriminately. It is a form of child abuse in animal society.

In contrast, if the animal mother and her offspring are together for the first four days of its life—the "sensitive period"—and are then separated for several days and then reunited, the mother quickly resumes her protective role. An imprinting has previously occurred for her and for the infant.

In Dr. Klaus's study, the human mothers in both the extended contact and the control groups all returned in one month with their babies for examination, as requested. Each mother was interviewed as to the general health of her infant and her caretaking habits. Each was observed while a pediatrician examined her infant, and each was filmed while she fed her infant. During all three procedures, mothers' responses were scored.

Mothers in the extended contact group were more responsive to their infant's needs, more reluctant to leave him or her in the care of another, and more attentive during physical examination. They also showed greater sensitivity to the infant's cries and made greater efforts to soothe him or her. This study and others indicate that mothers do have a "sensitive period" immediately following childbirth. Their bodies and minds cry out to hold and cuddle their babies. Their consuming desire is for imprinting and mothering. Neonatal contact makes for a better future mother.[12]

A Father Can Enhance His Infant's Development

In 1972, while in the midst of studies at New York Hospital-Cornell Medical Center aimed at learning how very early life experiences affect the infant's subsequent emotional development, Dr. Lee Salk, a psychologist, who is the author of a number of books on child psychology, said, "A good father is a little bit of a mother." Dr. Salk believes and regrets that society has largely deprived fathers—and their children—the rewards of this role.

"You rarely see a father on the cover of a magazine holding a baby and looking happy," he said. That is because Americans tend to think of fathers as being background figures who enter the picture only when the child is older and needs to be punished or launched into some manly pursuit. This failure to get fathers physically and emotionally involved in the care of their children from the moment of birth may deprive children of realizing fully the potential with which they were born.[13]

The central core of Dr. Salk's research is the well-documented observation that babies who are understimulated do not develop as well as babies with adequate stimulation. And fathers are keystones in that developmental stimulation. They add to or take away from the child's chances of realizing his or her inborn potential. Nonparental participation in the infant's activities subtract from this potential and may lay the groundwork for future emotional problems unless counteracted.

Dr. Salk said the period immediately after birth is a critical one for both the parents and the baby. Keeping the mother and her infant as close together as possible immediately after birth, instead of separating them as now is done at many hospitals, is important.

Dr. Salk feels it may also be possible to enhance a child's learning ability by enriching the environment immediately after birth, through rocking the baby, music, and visual stimulation of various kinds. The father could provide all this.

"There are a number of critical periods in development which markedly affect the child's future. If he gets a good foundation at an early age, there's not a thing later in life that can shake him up," said Dr. Salk. In this way, he believes, it will be possible to prevent many of the emotional problems which trouble children because the positive influences of things like early contact with mother and the early involvement of the father have not been fully appreciated.[14]

The Process of Parent-Infant Attachment

For a full clarification of bonding between a parent and his or her child, we went to Constance H. Keefer, M.D., a pediatrician who has made parent-infant bonding her specialty. She is a staff member of the Child Development Unit, Children's Hospital Medical Center of Boston. Dr. Keefer said, "I prefer the term *attachment* rather than *bonding* because *attachment* carries the meaning of a parent and a child getting to know each other—a process—which takes time, probably several years.

"Attachment includes certain elements. The child and parent know, love, and trust each other. It isn't new but is something accepted instinctively by parents since the beginning of mankind. Of late, however, parent-infant attachment has become a 'hot' issue in pediatrics. The critical issue in this whole area is the role of the medical professional in child development. The parental function must not be usurped by the professional," said Dr. Keefer.

In their book, *Maternal-Infant Bonding*, the two main authorities on the subject, Marshall H. Klaus, M.D., and John H. Kennell, M.D., a co-worker with Dr. Klaus at the same institutions, put forth seven principles that are crucial components in the process of parental attachment.[15] They are:

1. The "sensitive period"—the first minutes and hours of life, which we have described already. The coauthors reaffirm that it is necessary for the mother and father to have close contact with their neonate for later development to be optimal.
2. The species-specific responses to the infant by a mother and a father.

3. Only one infant at a time becomes attached optimally. That is to say, twins or triplets will become attached to their parents, but to one more than to another, and vice versa. This is called *monotropy*.

4. The mother's attachment to her infant is greater if there is some infant response such as body or eye movements. Drs. Klaus and Kennell admit, "You can't love a dishrag."

5. Witnesses to the birth process become strongly attached to the infant.

6. Some adults cannot go through the processes of attachment and detachment simultaneously. For example, a father may not be able to attach to his newborn while mourning the loss or threatened loss of his wife.

7. Early events have long-lasting effects. For instance, anxiety about the well-being of a sick newborn may cast long shadows and adversely shape the development of that child.

Like Parents, the Baby Prepares for Attachment

Dr. Keefer told us: "At this point it is only speculation in pediatrics, but we think that the baby along with the parents is preparing for attachment before birth. An infant in utero can hear. Sounds get through; the fetus responds to sound; and the mother's voice transmits readily through her diaphragm. The infant in utero becomes used to some aspects of his mother: her voice, heart rate, sleep-wake cycle, and her various moods. Obviously, then, the baby is not going to have to come out and start anew. He has a good idea of what his mother is like already and is prepared to attach to this familiar person.

"Once he is born," added Dr. Keefer, "the infant will show some clearly defined personality traits. He is not a mere lump of clay to be molded entirely. The child shows how he must be handled—clues are offered by quietude or crying. Additionally, he is able to learn a lot about his parents in the first days and weeks of life.

"From the first minutes, he can see and fix his eyes on what he wants to see, and in a few weeks will turn in the direction of his mother's face preferentially. His hearing capacity allows him to learn about his parents in the same way they learn about him. He turns sooner to a female voice as opposed to a male voice. And he responds to smell, indicated by a breast-fed baby who will respond preferentially to the odor of a breast pad with his own mother's milk on it as opposed to a breast pad with the milk of another lactating mother on it," she said.

These sentitivities of the newborn are well illustrated in a film made by Drs. Klaus and Kennell called *The Amazing Newborn*. It shows infants moving their limbs in time with the cadence and rhythms of parental speech, even opening the mouth to speak by those rhythms when only weeks old. Dr. Keefer showed us films also, which indicated interpersonal response of infants to their mothers.

"My message is that bonding is desirable during the first few minutes and hours of life, but it is not mandatory. A mother and father can make up for the lack of immediate bonding by the use of quality time later on. Immediate bonding is not a critical issue that must be achieved," said Dr. Keefer. "Attachment occurs firmly by interpersonal communication between the parent and the child over a long period."

However, Dr. Klaus and Dr. Kennell say: "This original mother-infant bond is the wellspring for all the infant's subsequent attachments and is the formative relationship in the course of which the child develops a sense of himself. Throughout his lifetime the strength and character of this attachment will influence the quality of all future bonds to other individuals."[16]

NOTES FOR CHAPTER TWENTY-ONE

1. Marshall H. Klaus and John H. Kennell, "Mothers Separated from Their Newborn Infants," *Pediatric Clinics of North America* 17:1015–37 (1970).

2. Susan Heller Anderson, "A Plea for Gentleness to the Newborn," *The New York Times*, January 15, 1978.

3. Anderson, "A Plea."

4. L. Gardner, "Deprivation Dwarfism," *Scientific American* 13:101–6 (1972).

5. L. Ourth and K. Brown, "Inadequate Mothering and Disturbance in the Neonatal Period," *Child Development* 32:287–95 (1961).

6. Ruth D. Rice, "Neurophysiological Development in Premature Infants Following Stimulation," *Developmental Psychology* 13:69–76 (1977).

7. Anderson, "A Plea."

8. Klaus et al., "Mothers Separated."

9. K. Robson, "The Role of Eye-to-Eye Contact in Maternal-Infant Attachment," *Journal of Child Psychology and Psychiatry* 8:13–25 (1967).

10. R. Rubin, "Maternal Touch," *Nursing Outlook* 11:828 (1963).

11. "Extended Neonate Contact Makes for Better Mother," *Obstetric and Gynecology News,* July 1, 1971.

12. Rice, "Neurophysiological Development."

13. Harry Nelson, "Early Role for Fathers in Care of Babies Urged," *Los Angeles Times,* June 15, 1972.

14. Nelson, "Early Role."

15. Marshall H. Klaus and John H. Kennell, *Maternal-Infant Bonding* (St. Louis: C. V. Mosby, 1976).

16. Klaus and Kennell, *Maternal-Infant Bonding.*

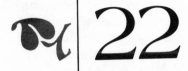

22

Factors for and Against Cesarean Section

The ideal incidence of abdominal delivery would be difficult to establish. The institution in which too few cesareans are done penalizes many mothers by the increasing frequency of extensive soft tissue damage and a higher incidence of babies who are born dead or . . . severely injured. . . . Too many cesareans substitutes a grossly artificial method for the normal physiologic reproductive mechanism.
—M. E. DAVIS, M.D., "The Modern Role of Cesarean Section," *Surgical Clinics of North America*

Brazilian Women and Obstetricians Prefer Cesarean Births

Natural prepared childbirth has increased in this country due to its many advocates among American women and American obstetricians. That is not the case in Brazil. There, most well-to-do women and their doctors prefer cesarean section performed at their option—simply a birth of convenience. In private Brazilian clinics, 60 percent of all deliveries are cesarean, although considered unethical and even illegal when not done for medical reasons.[1]

The Brazilian women choose cesarean birth because of widespread fears of the pain of childbirth or because of general misinformation that normal deliveries can lead to permanent vaginal and uterine deformities. One twenty-eight-year-old social assistant, Elaine Sadicoff, said she had chosen cesarean delivery because "some friends warned me that a normal childbirth would leave me internally deformed as far as sexual activity."

Brazilian obstetricians encourage the practice because it is lucrative. A normal delivery at a private clinic costs an average of $600, while a doctor often collects up to $1400 for a cesarean. "A substantial number of physicians in Brazil believe that the surgical delivery is the best method of childbirth—it causes no harm to the figure, it is quick, and it is a lot more profitable," said Paulo Belfort de Agular, M.D., the former president of the Brazilian Federation of Gynecology and Obstetrics Associations.[2]

"Many urban families today don't want more than two or three children, and women don't want to take contraceptive pills all their lives. So they take advantage of cesarean surgery and then have their fallopian tubes tied," Dr. Agular said.

On the other hand, some government medical authorities in Brazil have spoken out against the growing incidence of cesarean deliveries. João Yunes, M.D., a Health Ministry official and strong supporter of normal deliveries, lashed out at the private Brazilian medical system for embarking on an expensive public relations campaign in support of cesarean sections. In contrast to the 60 percent incidence in private Brazilian clinics, the frequency of cesarean operations at most state-run institutions is only about 10 percent. This still contrasts with World Health Organization estimates that worldwide only four of every hundred deliveries are cesarean.[3]

The Incidence of Cesarean Operation in the United States

As possibly shocking as Brazilian private clinic birth figures may be, the incidence of cesarean operations in the United States is not that far behind. The last several years have seen an increasing ratio of such deliveries to normal vaginal childbirths. From May 1975 through May 1976 there were 3,130,000 live births recorded in this country by the National Center for Health Statistics.[4] This is an estimated annual rate of 14.6 births per 1000 of the population—approximately 8575 new American mothers each day. The number of these mothers delivering by cesarean section "has grown from a 3–4 percent rate to 10–15 percent in the last five years, with reports of 30 percent in some areas," said Dr. B. Cochran in a 1974 report to the International Childbirth Education Association.[5]

For clarification, Dr. Cochran's statement of 30 percent of births performed by cesarean operation relates to hospitals dealing with high-risk patients such as women with diabetes.

The incidence of cesarean section has continued to climb as the use of technological advances constantly indicates more accurately which fetuses are at risk and can be delivered more safely surgically. We see, therefore, that the incidence of birthing by vaginal induction (see the next chapter) is decreasing, while the two methods at opposite ends of the childbirth spectrum, natural childbirth and cesarean deliveries, are increasing in the United States.

The Medical Indications for Cesarean Birth

In a cesarean section, an incision is made through the abdomen and into the uterus. The baby is lifted out and, usually, the placenta is also manually removed. It is done most frequently because the baby is too large to fit through the mother's pelvis (cephalopelvic disproportion) or is in a bad position causing dysfunctional labor. The baby may be overly big or the mother's pelvis really small.

The second most common problem that indicates a medical need for cesarean section is abnormal bleeding near the end of pregnancy. This might arise from the placenta lying in front of the baby's head, which we have described previously as *placenta previa*; or because the placenta has separated from its attachments on the uterus too early, *placental abruption*. The placenta previa requires an abdominal operation because the placenta would have to separate before the baby could come out. This would produce profound hemorrhage in the mother. Since the placenta is partially separating in placental abruption, this could cause the baby to no longer be supplied with oxygen and it would die from asphyxiation.

Another indication for birth by surgical operation is a fetus who is in any type of abnormal situation—either the breech positions we have described, a sideways position, or coming down face first instead of the back of the head first. Most abnormal presentations of fetuses are now delivered by cesarean section.

Up to now the least frequent indication for cesarean birth has been so-called "fetal distress," where the baby is not being well enough oxygenated either by the entanglement of the cord or insufficient functioning of the placenta. Nevertheless, Ervin E. Nichols, M.D., director of practice activities at the American College of Obstetricians and Gynecologists, said that more sophisticated methods of recognizing fetal distress, including a fetus-monitoring machine, is making this a more common reason for surgical intervention.

Finally, approximately 45 percent of American cesareans are due to a previous infant having been delivered surgically. It is the presence of a cesarean section scar or prior pelvic surgery, such as for urinary incontinence repair, that creates a problem. The dictum among doctors is "once a cesarean section, always a cesarean section," because of concern about the possibility of uterine rupture and its attendant hazards to both the mother and her unborn infant.[6,7,8,9]

The technique of accomplishing a cesarean section from an anatomic viewpoint, showing the placement of incisions and the liftout of the newborn is illustrated in Figures 41 through 50.

Starting with Figure 41, we see that an incision has been made across the woman's abdomen and low down just above her pubic hairline.

Figure 42 shows the scalpel cutting through the layer of the anterior rectus fascia surrounding the abdominal cavity.

Figure 43 shows the surgeon's fingers on the left elevating and separating the fascia from the rectus muscle. And in Figure 44 the peritoneum is vertically incised so that the surgeon can enter the peritoneal cavity. Once this is done, the operating table is tilted head down so that the front of the uterine wall is more or less horizontal. The patient is lying in what's known as the "Trendelenburg" position. The bowel drops away from the lower abdomen when the patient is placed in this position.

In Figure 45 the fold separating the bladder from the uterus is identified (the vesicouterine fold), doubly grasped and elevated in the midline. In Figure 46 it is cut with a short transverse incision made between the elevating thumb forceps and blunt dissection is carried out.

In Figure 47 a short transverse incision is made in the lower segment and in Figure 48 the incision is enlarged by the surgeon's fingers splitting of muscle fibers.

Figures 49 and 50 show the surgeon inserting a Murless extractor below the fetal head and delivering the baby out of the uterus.

Reasons for Planned Cesarean Delivery

There are three groups of basic reasons for elective cesarean delivery—all of them medically motivated. Vaginal birth may be desirable but dangerous if any of the following conditions are present in the mother or the fetus:

Some *pathological alteration* in the mother's body prior to or during pregnancy may make it highly undesirable to deliver vaginally, such as diabetes, chronic high blood pressure, or chronic kidney or

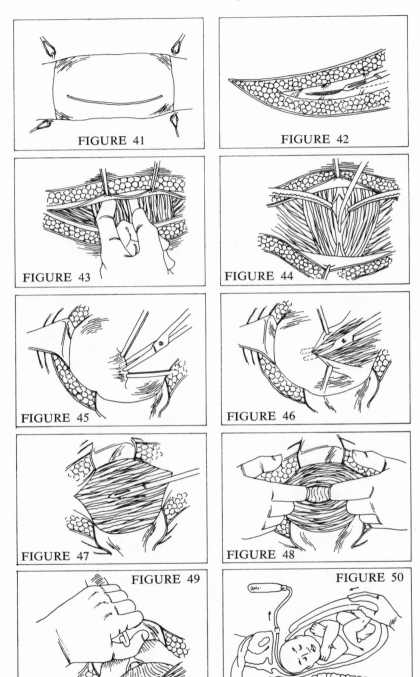

FIGURE 41

FIGURE 42

FIGURE 43

FIGURE 44

FIGURE 45

FIGURE 46

FIGURE 47

FIGURE 48

FIGURE 49

FIGURE 50

cardiac disease. In the best interest of fetus and parent, it may be the doctor's judgment that pregnancy termination by cesarean section be carried out at a preplanned time.

Sometimes there is an *Rh incompatibility* between the fetus and the mother, which could result in distress of the newborn or other babies to come later. This is a factor of fetal origin. An additional circumstance would be a prolapsed cord, that is the presentation of part of the umbilical cord ahead of the fetus with its compression between the fetus and the maternal pelvis.

The third basic group of reasons for cesarean section originate with either the mother or fetus, where a *mechanical interference* occurs with dilation of the cervix and/or expulsion of the fetus. Among the problems mentioned earlier were cephalopelvic disproportion, a bad position or poor presentation of the fetus; an overly large or malformed fetus; twins locked together; and uterine dysfunction or inertia.

When an individual's medical history indicates that a cesarean birth would be safer for the mother or child, an elective operation should be planned in advance. The labor process can be avoided. There is hardly an obstetric complication which has not been treated by cesarean section. It has come to be recognized as "one of the most dramatic procedures in the armamentarium of the surgeon."[10]

Risks Involved with the Cesarean Operation

While it was not always that way, in present-day obstetrics cesarean section is safe for mother and baby. The mortality from such an operation performed in the nineteenth century had been nearly 100 percent; today, it is less than 0.2 percent. But illness and death rates still remain higher for cesarean delivery than those associated with vaginal delivery.[11] Performing a cesarean is a major surgical act, with the inherent risks of anesthesia, shock, and hemorrhage.

Among the rare causes of maternal death resulting from cesarean section are inhalation anesthesia, blood transfusion reactions, pulmonary embolism, toxemia, and airlessness of the lungs due to failure of expansion or resorption of air from the alveoli. Between the two, the patient who is allowed a trial of labor before the surgery and the woman who undergoes an elective cesarean procedure, the laboring woman will be more in jeopardy.[12,13]

Risks are also involved following the cesarean operation, as well. Illness can occur from respiratory tract infection, urinary tract infection, genital tract infection, a bursting open of the wound, and the breaking off of an embolism from a blood clot.[14] There is more difficulty in curing infections because of prolonged labor with ruptured membranes and then cesarean section performed as an emergency procedure. Such an emergency situation adds to the surgical risk.

The Psychological Obstacle to Maternal-Infant Bonding

In 1953, D. Prugh, M.D., made some sensitive and insightful observations of mothers delivered of premature infants. He saw that the mother, particularly if the preemie is her first child, "often finds herself the prey of disturbing, and at times strongly conflicting feelings." Anxiety and guilt were the two most evident emotions he saw in the mother. She feared that something that she did or did not do during pregnancy affected the baby and produced the prematurity (and subsequent cesarean delivery).[15] Her thought was that some complication of prematurity produced a medical judgment that cesarean section was necessary, and so it took place.

In fact, many women feel a shame and guilt that the necessary operation, emergency or elective, is all their fault. Jini Fairley, who underwent a cesarean, expressed the common feeling: "I should have been more relaxed," or "If only I had gone to bed two weeks before . . ."[16]

Psychological obstacles to maternal-infant bonding are understandable. The cesarean-section patient has her baby taken from her, delivered without her participation or her husband's. If she has general anesthesia, it may be hours before she knows even the sex of her child. Medication and anesthesia blur memory and perception, leaving incomplete or perhaps false impressions that will linger in her memory all her life.

For those reasons, a number of cesarean support groups are forming around the country.

Parents Organize for Combating the Guilt of Cesarean Birth

When Nancy Cohen and her husband, Paul, went through prepared childbirth classes in 1972, they were anticipating the unique experience of birthing their baby. Unfortunately, a cesarean section was necessary instead. The baby, a boy, was born healthy, and both parents were grateful, but they knew they had missed one of life's great events. Nancy Cohen felt let down, depressed; she felt she had failed.

Her letter describing her feelings was published in the prepared childbirth newsletter, and a tremendous influx of responding letters arrived from other women feeling the same. Many women telephoned.

They did not repeat the shopworn phrase that mothers who experience cesarean section grow weary of hearing: "But you have a beautiful baby!"

Husbands feel the great disappointments and guilt as well. When their wives need them most, they are asked to leave, and can do nothing about giving support.

Mrs. Cohen and Mrs. Jini Fairley organized C/Sec—Caesarean/ Support, Education and Concern. By March 1977 C/Sec had amassed three thousand members and had helped eighty other such organizations to get started. C/Sec-type groups are located all over the nation as separate and autonomous organizations.

At C/Sec meetings, women, and sometimes, their husbands, speak of their experiences. Some women who had been well informed by their doctors and had received support from hospital staffs have reported good positive experiences. Others feel they have had bad experiences and feel a need to talk about them. A number believe they were routinely and unnecessarily separated from their babies. Their complaints are that nursing staffs were insensitive to their needs and treated them as extra work. A few mothers are really angry with their physicians. The mothers felt unprepared, uninformed, unsure of which questions to ask, and surprised at standard operating procedures. Many had gone on tours of delivery rooms, but were unfamiliar with operating rooms. When attached by tubes to intravenous fluids and catheterized, many women did not know what was happening and panicked. Some were offended repeatedly by the remarks of friends who imply that cesareans are chic, or that they are lucky to have escaped labor.

C/Sec cofounder, Nancy Cohen, related: "People would say, 'What's the difference? You got the easy way out. You will never have to go through labor.' Number one, it's not the easy way out. It's major surgery. Number two, I wanted to go through labor. I felt my baby should have a say in when he was born."[17]

If you would like to receive information about a cesarean birth support group in your area, contact the C/Sec organization, Caesarean/Support, Education and Concern, 15 Maynard Road, Dedham, Massachusetts 02026.

The Husband Gains a Role in Cesarean Birth

In a departure from traditional medical practice, Joseph O'Connor stayed by his wife, Carol Ann, as she underwent cesarean section at Terrace Heights Hospital in Hollis, Queens, New York, the morning of August 17, 1976. He was playing a supportive role in the cesarean delivery as husbands frequently do in natural, prepared childbirth. Gerald S. Stober, M.D., director of obstetrics and gynecology at Terrace Heights Hospital, screened the O'Connor family before selecting them to initiate the practice of allowing husbands to gain a role in cesarean birth at the hospital. Mrs. O'Connor gave birth to a healthy son, John Joseph.

"Actually the outcome of cesarean section is more predictable than with vaginal delivery. And so it's somewhat paradoxical to permit husbands to be present during vaginal delivery and not for cesarean." Said Dr. Stober. He stressed, however, that it is not appropriate for all couples. "You have to properly screen your patients."

Referring to Carol Ann O'Connor, the obstetrician said, "This woman is very well educated. The couple took the course in natural childbirth. They are not starry-eyed kids looking for an adventure. But they have certain psychological needs and we responded to them.

"For some time now the profession has experimented with fathers being in the delivery room for normal vaginal delivery. So this is broadening it for people who are properly prepared. We can say to people who are candidates for cesarean section that they do not have to be excluded from a meaningful birth experience."[18]

Nancy Lee Krauter underwent a cesarean section at Terrace Heights Hospital a year before Mrs. O'Connor, and her husband was not allowed to play a supportive role in the cesarean delivery as fathers do in prepared childbirth. She did some research and learned that Boston Hospital for Women allow the husbands of some women to be with their wives during the operation.

Mrs. Krauter founded the Caesarean Birth Association to serve as a source of information and reassurance for men and women facing cesarean delivery. To glean information on how to gain a role for husbands in your community hospital, contact the Caesarean Birth Association, Nancy Lee Krauter, coordinator, 125 North Twelfth Street, New Hyde Park, New York 11040. Telephone: (212) 523-8991.

Other cesarean support groups are:

Caesarean Support Group of New Jersey, Janet Keymetian, director, 184 Elm Avenue, Teaneck, New Jersey 07066. Telephone: (201) 692-9028.

Westchester ASPO, Prepared Caesarean Parents Committee, Box 125, Scarborough, Briarcliff Manor, New York 10510. Telephone: (914) 962-7696.

Mid-Hudson ASPO, Caesarean Parents Committee, Box 506, Fishkill, New York 12524. Telephone: (914) 225-6548.

Caesarean Concern Group, Debbie Carello, coordinator, 79 Putnam Street, Bristol, Connecticut 06010. Telephone: (203) 589-0674.

Caesareans for Sharing & Caring, Janet Taylor, director, 14 Top-stone Drive, Danbury, Connecticut 06810. Telephone: (203) 743-7344.

NOTES FOR CHAPTER TWENTY-TWO

1. "For Those Who Can Afford Them, Brazilian Women Prefer Cae-sarean Births," *The New York Times,* January 2, 1977.

2. *Times,* "Brazilian Women."

3. *Times,* "Brazilian Women."

4. *Monthly Vital Statistics Report* 25(5): 1 (1976).

5. B. Cochran, "Caesarean Section," in *Parent's Guide to the Child-bearing Year,* ed. P. Beals (Milwaukee, Wisconsin: The International Childbirth Education Association, 1974).

6. S. L. Romney et al., *Gynecology and Obstetrics: The Health Care of Women* (New York: McGraw-Hill, A Blakiston Publication, 1975).

7. M. E. Davis, "The Modern Role of Cesarean Section," *Surgical Clin-ics of North America* 33:101–23 (February 1953).

8. N. J. Eastman and L. M. Hellman (eds.), *William's Obstetrics* (New York: Appleton-Century-Crofts, 1971).

9. L. O. S. Poidevin, *Caesarean Section Scars* (Springfield, Ill.: Charles C Thomas, 1965).

10. H. P. Lattuada, "The Management of the Near-Term Pregnant Woman Who Dies Undelivered," *Clinical Obstetrics and Gynecology* 2(4): 1043–48 (December 1959).

11. H. L. Woodward et al., *Obstetric Management and Nursing* 6th ed. (Philadelphia: F. A. Davis, 1959).

12. E. W. Page, C. A. Villee, and D. B. Villee, *Human Reproduction: The Core Content of Obstetrics, Gynecology and Perinatal Medicine* (Phil-adelphia: W. B. Saunders, 1972).

13. J. J. Bonica, *Principles and Practice of Obstetric Analgesia and Anesthesia* (Philadelphia: F. A. Davis, 1972), vol. 2, *Clinical Considera-tions.*

14. J. R. Sutherst and B. D. Case, "Caesarean Section and Its Place in the Active Approach to Delivery," *Clinical Obstetrics and Gynecology* 2(1):241–61 (April 1975).

15. D. Prugh, "Emotional Problems of Premature Infants' Parents," *Nursing Outlook* 1:461–64 (1953).

16. Dee Wedemeyer, "Mothers Organizing to Combat the Guilt of Cae-sarean Birth," *The New York Times,* March 28, 1977.

17. *Times,* "Mothers Organizing."

18. Olive Evans, "Caesarean: A Husband Plays Role," *The New York Times,* August 18, 1976.

23

Labor Induction, Episiotomy, the Forceps, and Other Techniques in Modern Obstetrics

My bag of water broke at 1:05 P.M. Friday. I called my doctor, Parke Gray, and went to his office. After examining me, he sent me to the hospital directly where I arrived at 2:15 P.M. Very mild contractions started twenty-five minutes later. I didn't need to use any breathing techniques until 5:30 P.M. when I went into slow chest inhalations. Strong contractions began about an hour later, and I began my pant. I continued panting until I had the urge to push—around 10:00 P.M. I called the nurse who said I was fully dilated and could start pushing hard, probably to have the baby within the next half hour.

At 10:30 P.M., however, there still was no sign of my baby's head. Dr. Gray found that the baby's head had not rotated properly and faced toward the side, preventing it from dropping through the birth canal. As I had a contraction, he tried to turn the head with his hand. Finally, my

*obstetrician did it, but the shoulders wouldn't
turn. By this time, 12:30 P.M., I felt very weak
and tired. Dr. Gray recognized that. He decided
to move me into the delivery room to use the
suction device, a vacuum extractor, with which to
pull on the baby's head more efficiently. It was
working well and with a couple of good pushes, I
was able to move my child down and out of my
birth canal. Eli Scott Koster weighed 7 lbs.
10½ ozs. and was 20½ in. long when he was
born at 1:00 A.M., Saturday May 8, 1977.*
—MONICA L. KOSTER

The Elective Induction of Labor

Because her grandma was scheduled to visit this week to take care of the newborn, Agnes Brinkerhoff cajoled her doctor to induce labor. But the baby was not due for ten days and her obstetrician refused.

Labor brought on by artificial means before nature has a chance to act can be accomplished at the option of the physician. In modern obstetrics, more often than not the doctor's inclination is not to elect induction of labor unless medically required. In some instances it is as simple as rupturing the membranes surrounding the fetus.

Heretofore, elective inductions were performed simply for the mother's or obstetrician's convenience. We have suggested a reason that Agnes Brinkerhoff wanted an earlier delivery, but what about the doctor's reasons, if he had acquiesced? Before today, when the induced management of pregnancy is frowned upon by an obstetrician's peers, the doctor may have had a personal motivation for pushing along labor. Maybe he wished to play golf on the weekend and induced the woman's labor to get her off his mind. The practice carried a small but significant risk.

Roberto Caldeyro-Barcia, M.D., director of the Latin-American Center for Perinatology and Human Development and past president of the International Federation of Gynecologists and Obstetricians, said, "In the last forty years, many artificial practices have been introduced which have changed labor from a physiological event to a very complicated medical procedure in which unnecessary drugs and maneuvers are used, many of which are potentially damaging for the baby and for the mother."[1]

Therefore, since the choice to induce labor is not without complications, it should not be done for social convenience. Just because grandma is available now and not later is not a good enough reason for Agnes to want to speed her baby's birth date.

Unfortunately, even now there are some doctors and some hospitals who advocate elective induction of labor. Their argument is that if deliveries take place during the normal working hours then there can be an adequate staff provided in the obstetrical suite to cope with the patients. They also say that the nurses and the doctors are more awake, alert, and functioning. They are at their best during the day. The woman, too, is better able to accept labor because she has had a good night's sleep prior to labor inducement. Relaxation and rest help labor along.

We do not agree with these arguments, valid as they may sound. The fact is that nature causes babies to come at random. On the average, as many babies are born at three o'clock in the afternoon as are born at three o'clock in the morning. Labor is not supposed to follow an eight-hour working day, and we feel strongly that elective induction is an interference in the natural process that heightens the risk of morbidity to the child.

If carried to the extreme of every pregnant woman being induced during the normal working hours, a disproportionate number of non-mature children will result. Furthermore, labor contractions will be too strong, or too prolonged, or too difficult for the infant and for the mother. The potential for abuse is too great. So we do not advocate—in fact, we deplore—the elective induction of labor.

An editorial in the prestigious British medical journal, *The Lancet*, published in November 1974, and brought to our attention by an article in *The New York Times*, said: "Induction on the grounds of social convenience is a pernicious practice which has no place in modern obstetric care. The mother's holiday, the calls of the obstetrician's private practice, must not influence for the sake of even a few days, an event which for the child may affect the outcome of its entire life."[2]

An Instance of Medical Indication for Labor Induction

Of course, there are medical indications for labor induction. If the child is past due or membranes have ruptured in the latent stage before the labor onset and it seemed not to be coming on, then induction would be called for. And other valid medical reasons such as the mother's affliction with toxemia, diabetes, or high blood pressure are the only kinds allowed. Induced labor is part of modern obstetrical care for the purpose of unburdening the term of pregnancy.

Being two weeks overdue for the birth of her second child, Ingrid Casolo was examined by her obstetrician who found that most of the amniotic fluid had been resorbed from her uterus. The doctor's fingers felt only the uterus around the fetus without any fluid present, a confirmation that she was indeed postmature. Her cervix was four centimeters dilated, even though she was not laboring. On-and-off cramping for a few days was felt by the woman, but nothing more.

The circumstance of postmaturity on the part of the baby was a strong medical indication for induction of labor. The thinning of the mother's cervix and partial dilation was characteristic of an easy potential induction.

The obstetrician admitted his patient to the hospital at 11:30 A.M., where she was prepared, had an enema, and received a slow intravenous infusion of oxytocin. *Oxytocin* is a hormone elaborated by the pituitary gland. It functions to make the uterus contract. Pure oxytocin, synthesized in the laboratory (Pitocin), is readily available. When properly administered, synthetic oxytocin is almost 100 percent certain to bring about the onset of labor.

Within a half hour Ingrid Casolo was contracting regularly, and her physician ruptured her membranes. Further confirming his initial impression of postmaturity, he found no fluid in her uterus. She progressed rapidly so that three hours after rupturing the membranes the young woman had a normal delivery of a healthy baby girl, whom she and her husband named Sandi.

Upon being interviewed at the hospital two days later, Mrs. Casolo said, "The doctor induced me at two P.M.; the labor started shortly after, and I began pushing about forty-five minutes after that. The delivery came fast—I enjoyed it! It was different from my first-time birth, when it was terrible—really long and hard. Even Demerol did not help then. This second time, it was easy. I prefer the inducement. It was terrific!"

The Techniques of Labor Induction

The earliest form of labor induction consisted simply in giving the mother a large, hot enema or having her take castor oil. Stimulation of the bowel by these means sometimes carried over into labor. Indeed, many obstetricians and midwives still use the enema means of stimulation. Once contraction of the uterus starts, it usually continues. If the uterus is not ready to contract, these procedures will not work.

As illustrated with Ingrid Casolo, a woman with delayed labor is given oxytocin to start contractions. The intravenous infusion is easily controllable. An infusion pump carefully adjusts the oxytocin dose so that not more than one milliliter in twenty minutes is administered. This is a tiny amount, and the pump method of giving the drug is different than it used to be. Now, oxytocin administration is safer.

A woman who is in labor but whose uterine contractions are inadequate to effect delivery can also have her labor augmented by the oxytocin infusion technique. It is done after pelvic measurement to make sure the baby will fit through the birth canal. Feeling the bones of the pelvis inside through the vagina and assessing the size of the infant must be carried out with accuracy. Since the doctor is not always perfect with measurements, he or she may back up the assessment with X-ray examination. He or she compares the baby's head to the pelvic spread.

Peter A. Goodhue, M.D., an obstetrician-gynecologist and the practice partner of one of the authors, believes X-ray measurement of the mother's pelvic bones is a useful adjunct prior to induction of labor. "The doctor must make sure that the baby is going to fit through the pelvic opening," Dr. Goodhue said. "The X-radiation definitely does not affect the baby. This has been studied over forty years without any ill effects being noted. However, some obstetricians no longer use X-ray pelvimetry because they consider it of little value."

Risks Connected with Labor Induction by Drug Use

"In 1974, in New York City, a hundred and sixty babies were born following elective induction, weighing less than twenty-five hundred grams [about five and a half pounds, the medical definition of prematurity] and of those, twelve died," said Jean Pakter, M.D., the director of New York City's maternity and family-planning services in an address to the American Public Health Association, October 20, 1976. "Elective inductions which are primarily for the convenience of the physician and/or the expectant mother accounted for more than half the total of inductions citywide."

Dr. Pakter did a statistical analysis covering 1974 and 1975 and found that 80 percent of all induced deliveries with drugs were with middle-class, private patients. These women should have fewer complications in birth because of the excellence of private care, but they do not. "The question that remains unanswered," Dr. Pakter said, "is whether or not we are going to have average levels of prematurity and more fetal distress in a group of infants that should have the lowest risk of all babies born."[3]

Under drug induction, labor lasts for less than three hours. Less than one-sixth of noninduced labor is that quick. The reason for shorter labor in induced deliveries is that oxytocics cause contractions to come faster and stronger, speeding up the time of labor.

But scientific studies have shown that babies need the seconds between contractions to replenish oxygen and stabilize their breathing. Consequently, there may be fetal distress due to lack of oxygen and intracranial hemorrhage, and trauma may result from violent uterine contractions.

The report from a review of 3324 elective inductions of labor with drugs at the University of Pennsylvania Hospital stated: "Amniotomy carries with it the risk of injury to the mother or fetus and displacement of the presenting part, resulting in malposition, prolapsed cord, prolonged latent period and infection. The hazards of the use of oxytocin in labor are related directly to the dose for a given individual. Overdosage results in uterine spasm with possible separation of the placenta, tumultuous labor, amniotic fluid embolus, afibrinogeneimia, lacerations of the cervix and birth canal, postpartum hemorrhage and uterine rupture. There may be water intoxication due to the antidiuretic effect of oxytocin. . . . Fetal and/or maternal mortality are, of course, ever-present dangers."[4]

We repeat: we strongly recommend against any mother seeking the elective induction of labor through drugs. Our judgment is that the risks are too great unless there are medical necessities for its use.

Is Episiotomy Really Required for Delivery?

Over centuries of obstetrical care various techniques have been devised to make the birth process easier. The most frequent operative procedure is the *episiotomy*, a cut of the skin and muscles between the vagina and anus to enlarge the birth canal. Episiotomy prevents tears or lacerations of the tissue which generally occur during the course of delivery from the extreme stretching of the vagina. Tissue tears are jagged, do not follow anatomic lines, and are difficult to repair. They usually happen at the lowermost portion of the vagina because it could not stretch enough to fit over the baby's head. Most of the time, first babies delivered completely naturally without any interference will produce ragged tears. The poor functional healing of such tears can affect a woman's future sex life. In anticipation of this tissue tearing, a modern obstetrician makes a straight-line skin cut with scissors following anatomic lines to ensure healing without scarring.

The technique for performing the episiotomy from an anatomic viewpoint is shown in Figures 51 and 52. Figure 51 shows blanching of the tissues indicating the need for such a cut. It will prevent a jagged uneven laceration. A precise, clean-cut surgical incision heals better, repairs more readily, and gives a much more satisfactory result for the woman over a period of time.

Figure 51 also shows the lower birth canal almost completely distended by the baby's head. Dotted lines indicate the site of potential cuts. Straight down toward the anus is known as the "midline episiotomy" and does not include the fibers of the external sphincter ani muscle which surrounds the anal opening. Perpendicular to this midline cut is the lateral episiotomy shown by the dotted line off to the side.

Figure 52 shows the obstetrical surgeon making a right mediolateral episiotomy, which is midway between the other two at a 45-degree angle. Note that a protective blunt scissors is employed to make the straight incision rather than a scalpel. For the uncomplicated birth this incision is usually timed to coincide with the height of a uterine contraction when the perineum is well distended.

Repair of an episiotomy with sutures is deferred until after the placenta has separated and been expressed out of the birth canal by th new mother.

In pointing out obstetrical progress, Dr. Goodhue said, "Twenty or more years ago the most common episiotomy cut was made off to the side and into the buttock tissues, but this caused severe discomfort for the patient. The reason for this side cut was that midforceps deliveries were attempted before the perineum was much distended, thus preventing prolapsed uterus, herniation of the rectum or hernia of the bladder. Today, the sideways cut for episiotomy is seldom done because midforceps isn't attempted unless absolutely necessary. Instead a vertical cut with one snip is made from the lower part of the vaginal opening, down toward the anus.

"Now, women ask me all the time," continued Dr. Goodhue, "if I do episiotomies routinely. I usually do an episiotomy. But if the patient desires to try delivery without it, I will perform an episiotomy only if it looks like the vaginal tissue is going to tear. Blanching of the tissues is the clue. The obstetrician's judgment must be relied upon to decide whether or not an episiotomy is required at the time of delivery.

"It happens that thirty years ago the most common gynecological operation in this country was a repair of the vagina ten years after childbirth. The older woman's vagina was falling down or bulging out because of injury at the time of delivery. By the performance of episiotomy in modern obstetrics, this late sequelae of vaginal relaxation is eliminated for the woman years hence.

"In all honesty I must add that some women can deliver without an episiotomy. Tears will not occur for people with more elasticity of the tissues such as with ice skaters or ballet dancers. That type of athletic woman is not the norm," said Dr. Goodhue.

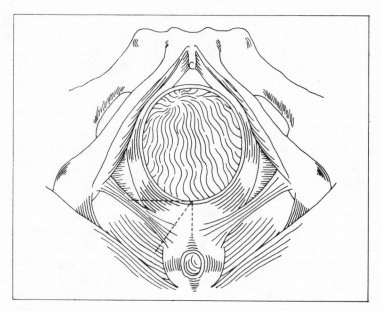

FIGURE 51

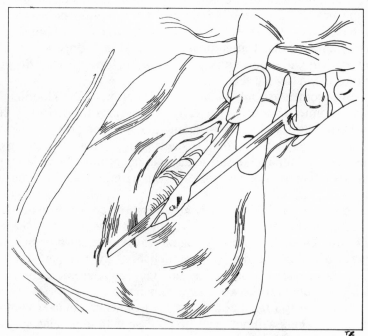

FIGURE 52

Episiotomy, Lax Vagina, and Your Sex Life

The main muscular support to the pelvic floor is the *levator ani muscle*, a broad muscle made up of several components. It stretches when the infant's head emerges. If overstretched and torn, the levator ani muscle gives less support to the back wall of the vagina where it is separated from the rectum. The bladder also loses support because it sits on this muscle when the woman is in an erect posture.

Over time, the bladder's weight pushes down on the levator ani muscle and lets the vaginal chamber grow wider than it should be. Such laxity causes a loss of sexual function, since the penis will plop around in this big vagina and provide less sexual sensation for both man and woman.

Furthermore, a lax vagina gives rise to less control over bladder function. There will be urine loss when the woman coughs, sneezes, or strains in some way. The strain puts stress on the bladder itself, and the muscle supposed to be holding it up has no power to perform its function anymore. Symptoms such as these will show among women with lax vaginas in the forty-, fifty-, or sixty-year age groups. Episiotomy at the time of childbirth saves the woman from these later symptoms, preventing overstretching of the levator ani muscle.

Along that line, Dr. Goodhue said, "We have patients who mention that their husbands don't find them as tight as they used to be before they had babies, and sexual intercourse is not being enjoyed as much by the husband. Knowing about this, a husband will jokingly say at the time of delivery, 'Put an extra stitch in for me!' The 'husband's stitch' is talked about in jest, but some husbands are partly serious. However, sexual counselors have told me that the 'husband stitch' has no validity. If there is a significant complaint about lack of sexual enjoyment, there may be some other underlying psychological problem."

The Use of Obstetrical Forceps for Ease of Delivery

An infant does not always slide down the birth canal with ease, popping into the doctor's outstretched hands. The baby can get stuck, since vaginal tissue is not all that stretchable. Obstetrical forceps, various-sized instruments frequently shaped like spoons, fit into the birth canal without causing injury to the mother. They were developed a few hundred years ago as a means of grasping the infant and lifting it out of the uterus.

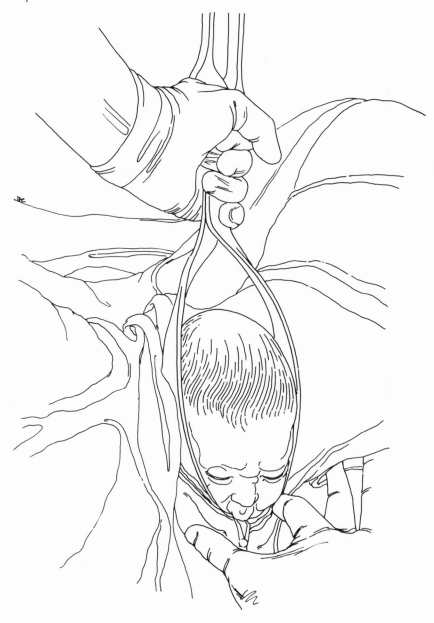

FIGURE 53

The spoon portions of the forceps fit around the baby's head and put their pressure on the cheekbones, the most highly developed part of the head. This prevents injury to the brain. Traction is applied over the cheekbones to bring the baby down the birth canal and to turn it as needed.

Forceps technique is complicated and requires skill that only comes with practice. Properly used, they are extremely safe for both baby and mother. If some kind of injury should occur from forceps use, it would be to the mother. It is very difficult to injure the baby with forceps. If brain damage occurred it would be due to the condition that called for the use of forceps rather than from the forceps themselves. The use of forceps is an operative procedure and requires anesthesia.

"In the last few years, young obstetricians have been getting less training in the use of forceps. Few of them have the opportunity to learn difficult operative obstetrics with the forceps instruments," said Dr. Goodhue. "Those difficult deliveries are much safer by cesarean section."

The Vacuum Extractor to Suck Out the Baby

Inasmuch as forceps take up room in the birth canal and cannot be applied to the head of just *any* stuck baby, suction cup devices of several types have been developed. The most successful one, the Malstrom Vacuum Extractor, was recently invented and was the one used for Monica L. Koster and described by her at the start of this chapter. It allows for the baby's scalp, which is quite loose, to be sucked without very great negative pressure. Damage to the baby is avoided and only a "chignon," which is an outpocketing of the scalp, forms temporarily. Signs of suction use are gone usually in a day or two.

The Malstrom Vacuum extractor is a round metal cup that is placed on the baby's head. At the other end, an apparatus that looks like a bicycle pump provides the negative pressure for suction. Figure 54 show the cup placed on the baby's head. At this point, the mother is fully dilated and pressure is built up sufficiently by the pump, the obstetrician pulls with suction on the infant's head each time a contraction occurs. Figure 55 shows the baby taken from the birth canal and the doctor detaching the round metal cup from the head. Natural delivery is aided this way when the woman is having a prolonged second stage of labor, and there is no injury to mother or child. No anesthesia is necessary for employment of the vacuum extractor. It is just another means for efficient delivery in modern obstetrics.

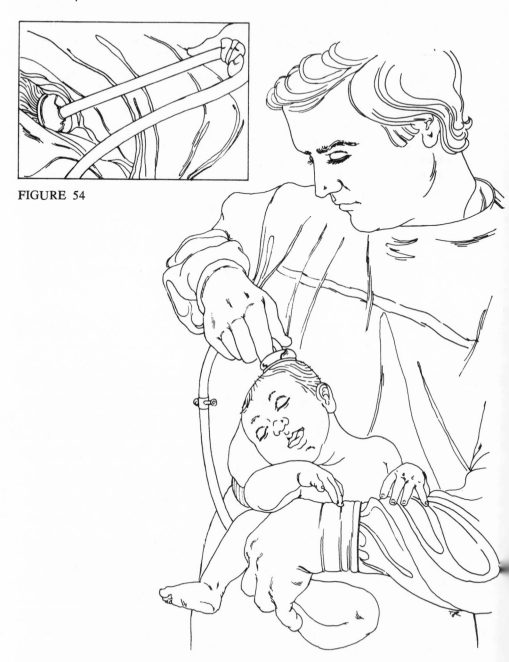

FIGURE 54

FIGURE 55

NOTES FOR CHAPTER TWENTY-THREE

1. Barbara Yuncker, "Delivery Procedures That Endanger a Baby's Life," *Good Housekeeping,* August 1975.

2. Jane E. Brody, "Some Obstetrical Methods Criticized," *The New York Times,* April 10, 1975.

3. Nancy Hicks, "Study Is Sought on the Practice and Safety of Drug-induced Births," *The New York Times,* October 24, 1976.

4. H. Fields, "Complications of Elective Induction," *Obstetrics and Gynecology,* 15:476–80 (1960).

24
Fetal Monitoring and Newborn Evaluation

While Sweden, Finland and the Netherlands compete for the honor of having the lowest incidence of infant deaths per one thousand live births (in the first year of life), the United States continues to find itself outranked by fourteen other developed countries. . . . In light of the fact that in most of the other listed countries there is no strong feeling of obligation to preserve life when a live birth results in extreme prematurity, severe congenital malformation or impairment, their incidence of infant mortality should be greater than ours, not less.
—DORIS B. HAIRE, D.M.S.,
The Cultural Warping of Childbirth

The Future of the Unborn Is Brighter Than Ever Before

Dramatic changes in childbirth are taking place in this century, and they are threefold. Already, motherhood has been made much less risky than ever before. Second, women are experiencing reduced discomfort from labor and delivery by childbirth preparation classes and with the use of anesthesia. Now obstetricians have undertaken the third advancement—to reduce dangers for the unborn while the mother is pregnant.

Developments in obstetrics in the last decade have been so phenomenal that the future of the unborn is brighter than ever before.

Their potential is to be healthy newborns 98.3 percent of the time. New discoveries and additional knowledge are making this possible.

This is not to say that well-established and valuable precepts should be shunted aside. "There is no substitute for early, continued, careful prenatal care, with strong emphasis on the health of the mother (both mental and physical). Proper nutrition, early diagnosis and vigorous treatment of any disease or health problem of the mother will help to avoid complications for the baby she is carrying," says Arnold Melnick, D.O., of Cheltenham, Pennsylvania, chief of pediatrics in nearby Delaware Valley Hospital and Parkview Hospital. Dr. Melnick is also editor of *Maternal and Child Health*, a medical journal.[1] We heartily agree with his statements.

Monitoring of the Fetus Before Labor

While a conscientious nurse and zealous doctor are still the best monitors of the condition of a laboring woman and her unborn child, there are some more recent technical developments in medicine which are useful adjuncts. The old means of monitoring the unborn have not been abandoned either.

The earliest form of fetal monitoring was simply listening to the baby's heartbeat in labor. The usual heart rate is 120 to 160 beats per minute. A significantly lower rate implied something was wrong— often, insufficient oxygen going to the fetus. While not disregarded, this form of monitoring is of limited value because states of chronic oxygen lack can exist without affecting the baby's heart rate until the last minute. More sophisticated methods of monitoring were searched for and perfected.

An antepartum test performed before labor observes the amniotic fluid which is normally clear. If a fetus is suffering distress at any time, it will move its bowels inside the uterus, passing stool (meconium). This will make the amniotic fluid discolor a brownish green, which can be observed by passing a small instrument through the cervix and using a strong light to see the cloudiness of the fluid. Additionally, fluid can be withdrawn through a needle into the amniotic sac—called *amniocentesis.*

The use of ultrasound to measure the size of the baby's head enables the obstetrician to predict the difficulty of the child's passage through the birth canal. This technique with the Doppler Ultrasound device is noninvasive and allows for two-dimensional motion studies. It is a "seeing" with sound. Sonar signals are transmitted, bounced off the fetus, and received back again to give a fetal picture. The unborn can be examined for an unlimited period of time. Ultrasound is free of radiation and has no known hazards.

Obstetricians also have means during labor for assessing the actual oxygen content of the fetus's blood and its acidity. In labor, with membranes ruptured, blood can be sampled. Methods have been devised to prick the scalp of the baby while it is still in the uterus and measure the chemical balance of its blood so the obstetrician is immediately alerted to the development of severe acidosis. *Blood acidosis* is an actual or relative decrease of alkali in proportion to the content of acid. Tissue function is often disturbed in this state, most importantly that of the central nervous system.

Additional forms of fetal monitoring occur with each visit to the obstetrician. The unborn infant is measured and charted in terms of its growth rate. The mother is weighed and questioned. As the time draws closer for delivery, more intense fetal monitoring is carried out. Abnormalities of pregnancy such as anemia, hypertension, diabetes, or pregnancy prolongation may require chemical testing of substances elaborated by the fetus.

Estriol, a hormone substance in the maternal urine, is known to have a specific concentration which is charted. A certain amount must be present, and if it is not, a problem with the fetus is recognized. As the baby and placenta get bigger, the estriol increases in the urine every few days. If it falls significantly, this indicates that the placenta is functioning inadequately, and the child's needs are not being met. This pregnancy will have to be terminated then, either by induction of labor or cesarean section. Therefore, the measurement of estriol by a special laboratory is an excellent noninvasive way to do fetal monitoring.

The Oxytocin Challenge Test

Another monitoring device determines how the infant's heart rate responds to artificially stimulated uterine contractions. *The oxytocin challenge test* involves administration of oxytocin and measurement of the uterine contractions and baby's heart rate simultaneously. A monitoring machine is attached to the mother. A normal fetal heartbeat indicates a healthy baby that can reside within the uterus for another week. Abnormality calls for quick delivery.

Procedure for the oxytocin challenge test includes recording the infant heart rate, giving a minimal dose of oxytocin by intravenous infusion to the mother, watching her uterus respond with regular contractions, and checking the fetal heart rate response. If the infant's heart rate slows down abnormally to the contractions, this is a positive oxytocin challenge test and indicates that the pregnancy should be ended.

It is fair to say that fetal monitoring using a monitoring machine is one of the most controversial aspects of modern obstetrics. There are doctors in this country who believe that every single labor should be monitored by machine. Proponents of home birth and others who want more natural delivery say that attaching these instruments to the mother is interfering in the true process of childbearing and is potentially harmful.

Our position on the subject is that we are not for *routine* fetal monitoring. But we do believe in the need for selected monitoring of problems in childbirth. Undoubtedly, any birthing attendant will feel more comfortable watching a woman with toxemia, or some other medical difficulty, if she is attached to a monitoring device. There is no question of its benefit. Babies have been saved by monitoring.

How a Fetal Life Was Saved by Monitoring

Phyllis and Baxter Franken were expecting their first child. Phyllis arrived at the hospital in labor at the same time that her physician was waiting for another of his patients to deliver. Both women labored in adjoining rooms simultaneously. The other woman was experiencing normal contractions and dilating fairly actively, while Phyllis Franken's fetus showed signs that it was in trouble. The unborn's heart rate tended to slow down each time a contraction came on, then it would come back up again. Because of this indication, the attending obstetrician attached this first-time mother to a fetal monitor.

When monitoring a fetus, this particular doctor makes it a practice to enlist the father's aid in watching his infant's progress. He teaches the father how to read the squiggles being drawn on graph paper by the monitoring machine. One function of the monitor is to measure the uterine contractions by a strain gauge placed on the mother's abdomen or by a pressure catheter placed directly into her uterus. In the case of Phyllis Franken, the external strain gauge was used. It consisted of a pair of belts, each with a small electronic sensor attached. Within seconds, Mr. and Mrs. Franken were able to watch two moving lines on a television-like box next to the bed. Graph paper slowly rolled out of the box's opening and a pattern of the baby's heartbeat was traced on it.

Baxter Franken observed the graph lines being drawn and periodically reported their readings to the obstetrician. The lines appeared normal each time the doctor asked. His other patient was ready to give birth and was taken into the delivery room. The obstetrician had just

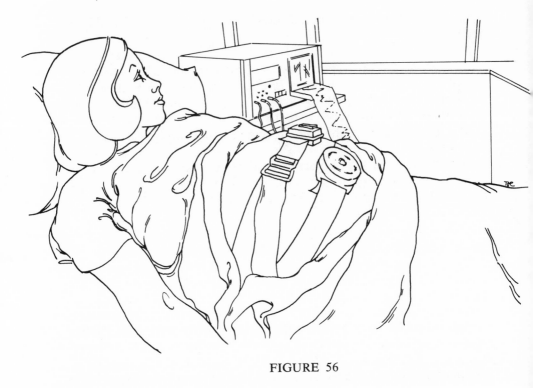

FIGURE 56

begun his sterile scrub when Baxter Franken came running from his wife's labor room, saying, "Hey, Doc, the pressure gauge is way up—very high now—and the baby's heart rate has slowed way down."

Immediately, the obstetrician called for a hospital resident physician to deliver his other patient and went tearing down the hall to Phyllis Franken. A quick glance at the graphs showed that this was indeed a life-threatening problem for the infant. The woman was fully dilated and could not keep from bearing down. Each time she pushed, the cord, which it turns out was wrapped around the baby's neck, was overstretched to cut off fetal oxygen. The baby had to be delivered fast, or it would die in minutes. Without the fetal monitoring device and the father reading it correctly, this would not have been known. The obstetrician was able to deliver the child alive.

The Nonstress Fetal Test

In studying fetal monitoring with the oxytocin challenge test, it was learned that fetuses are very much like people. When the fetus is active its heart rate speeds up, and when it is sleeping its heart rate slows down. A nonstress fetal test was developed that does not require intravenous injection of oxytocin.

The mother is attached to the monitor continuously, and when she feels her infant move inside of her she marks the graph at the spot recording the fetal heart rate at that moment. The infant's heart rate should have increased just then. This speedup indicates a healthy fetus —a simple test that takes twenty minutes and does not interfere with the pregnancy in any way. If the fetal heartbeats do not increase with internal movement noted by the mother, that indicates a problem with the unborn and other, more sophisticated monitoring may be undertaken.

Internal Monitoring of the Fetus

L. Stanley James, M.D., director of the division of perinatal medicine at the Columbia-Presbyterian Medical Center, New York City, foresees an increase in the use of monitoring "because there's so much it can tell us about what we need to know before labor and about how a baby is progressing during labor. We are, for instance, studying various types of movements of the head and chest in utero and relating them to abnormalities found afterward; we are developing ways of continuously measuring the fetal level of oxygen by means of a tiny electrode that works like an electrocardiograph, and we're working on ways of analyzing what's going on in the blood of both mother and baby during labor and following the relationship.

"The monitor provides us with a whole new horizon of information and techniques aimed at having the baby born in the best possible condition and making things more comfortable for the mother," Dr. James said. "As the technology is perfected, the monitors will become less obtrusive, more convenient for the mother."[2]

One of the more obtrusive and less convenient monitors is the apparatus that involves internal monitoring. It is used to assess accurately the infant's status during labor. A fine plastic catheter is placed into the uterus alongside the fetal head. (Of course, the membranes around the child have to be ruptured first.) Through the catheter, uterine contractions are measured in millimeters of mercury and traced on monitor paper, just as with external monitoring using the strain gauge.

Along with this internal catheter, a small electrode is attached to the baby's scalp to record the infant electrocardiogram and instantaneous heart rate. The monitoring machine integrates the distance on the cardiogram from one heartbeat to the next and prints this as beats per minute. By this method the baby's status can be determined at all times.

Internal fetal monitoring is a proper technique for use on any woman with some abnormality during pregnancy. Some authorities say it should be applied for every labor, because abnormalities of fetal heart rate can develop at any time during labor. As we have indicated, this recommendation is highly controversial. Risks do exist with internal fetal monitoring. An intrauterine catheter introduced over a long number of hours can provide an entry for infection. More problems may be created than it solves. Further, the monitoring machinery is extremely expensive and impossible to be furnished to every hospital.

We again say that we are opposed to routine internal fetal monitoring. It should only be employed when medically indicated.

Medical Evaluation of the Newborn

Historically, babies at birth are supposed to cry. One measurement of old midwives about the brightness of an infant was the time difference in cry from the moment of birth. A more valuable objective evaluation of the newborn is a system developed in 1953 by Virginia Apgar, M.D., an anesthesiologist, now deceased. *The Apgar score* is taken on the new baby at one minute after birth, disregarding expulsion of the cord and placenta. Measurements made are heart rate, respiratory effort, muscle tone, reflex irritability, and color.

- The infant's heart rate is graded over 100, under 100, or absent.
- A good cry, a weak cry, or no respiration is noted next.
- Observation is then made as to whether the muscle tone is actively flexing and moving or whether it is limp.
- The doctor determines if the baby cries upon being stimulated or only grimaces or remains limp: the test for reflex irritability.
- A color recording is checked as to the infant's pinkness all over, or the presence of blue extremities or a blue color all over.

These observations are given values of 2, 1, and 0, respectively; the higher number indicates greater health. All five evaluations are scored. The perfect Apgar score for a newborn is 10. One which is dead will be scored 0 (see Table 4).

If an infant scores 7 or better at one minute after birth, nothing need be done for it. A score between 3 and 6 at one minute demands oxygen and sucking out of the trachea. Scored 0 to 3, a newborn must have more intensive measures—visualization of trachea or vocal cords with a little instrument. A tube is passed to suck out secretions, and mouth-to-tube breathing is done at the same time cardiac massage is delivered. The delivery room personnel must work quickly to bring back the baby's vitality.

Five minutes after birth a second Apgar score is taken. This correlates with the future potential of the infant. If the score of 7 or better is not achieved by now, the baby has likelihood of having a neurological deficit at some future time.

Infants with an Apgar score of 0 have a 44 percent mortality rate during the first twenty-eight days of life compared to a neonatal mortality rate of 0.2 percent for babies with an Apgar score of 10. Babies with low scores are high-risk infants and often are kept under careful observation while in the nursery. Apgar score records have cast new light on many neonatal disturbances. The parents of newborns have every right to know their babies' Apgar scores, since this scoring may be indicative of how the child will progress into adulthood. Ask your doctor.

TABLE 4

Sign	0	1	2
Heart rate	absent	below 100	over 100
Respiratory effort	absent	slow, irregular	good, crying
Muscle tone	limp	some flexion of extremities	active motion
Reflex irritability	no response	grimace	cough, sneeze, or cry
Color	blue, pale	body pink, extremities blue	completely pink

Apgar scoring: Sixty seconds after completion of delivery of the infant the baby is scored from 0 to 2 on each of the five objective signs. A score of 10 (the highest possible score) indicates a baby in optimum condition. Neonatal mortality is inversely related to the Apgar score.

How the New Mother May Evaluate Her Newborn

Picture for yourself the delivery room activity and the new mother, awake and aware, observing what is going on around her. Only a few seconds have gone by since she delivered her baby. She is looking over the bulge of her abdomen; the infant has been placed there; amniotic fluid is running from its orifices. For a few minutes, the woman's obstetrician is doing nothing but observing the baby—perhaps massaging it. The suction apparatus is ready to aspirate fluids. In his head, the doctor is literally adding up the numbers of his Apgar scoring.

Suppose you are that new mother. What might you do to make your own evaluation of your newborn? We suggest an evaluative method for checking certain physical signs at once. Many hospitals have large charts on Apgar scoring posted in each delivery room so that all delivery room personnel become familiar with the method. We recommend that you can go into delivery with your own chart posted in your head and score your newborn yourself.

See that your baby is breathing normally. Most babies do not immediately cry at birth. While lying on the mother's abdomen, an infant will breathe quietly. Frequently he or she will open his or her eyes, even before the umbilical cord is clamped. Usually his head seems too big for the body. It may be nicely rounded or temporarily out of shape—lopsided or elongated due to pressure before or during birth. A bald head or a crop of thick hair are both normal.

The infant's eyes may have a blank, stary gaze, especially if drugs were involved in the birthing. The eyes will be colored blue or gray and one or both may turn to crossed to walleyed position. The eyelids may be puffy.

Don't let the face disappoint you, since many newborns look like little old men. They have pudgy cheeks, a broad flat nose with merely the hint of a bridge, a receding chin, and a slightly underslung jaw.

On the skull you will see or feel two soft spots or *fontanels*. There is one above the brow and another close to the crown of the head. The scalp skin may be loose and the brow wrinkled. Indeed, the skin over the rest of the body is thin and dry. You may see veins through it. Fair skin may be rosy-red temporarily, and downy hair is not unusual. Some white, prenatal skin covering called *vernix caseosa* may be coating his body.

Mothers often count the fingers and toes as the first thing. The hands, in fact, are usually held in a characteristic tight-fist position. When opened, they show finely lined palms, tissue-paper-thin nails, dry, loose-fitting skin, and deep bracelet wrist creases. The feet look more complete than they are. An X-ray examination would show only one real bone at the heel. Other bones are now cartilage. Skin on the feet is often loose and wrinkly.

Your baby's legs will most likely be drawn up against the abdomen in the prebirth position. When they are measured later, the extended legs will be shorter than you would expect compared to the length of the arms. The knees will stay slightly bent and the legs remain somewhat bowed for a while.

The newborn's whole body may startle you in some normal detail. For instance, you may see a short neck, small, sloping shoulders, swollen breasts, large rounded abdomen, an umbilical stump created from the doctor's cutting the cord, and a slender and narrow pelvis and hips. The genitals of both boys and girls will seem large in the newborn, in comparison to their overall size. The scrotal sac in baby boys is relatively large.

His color should be pink, with a deep flush spreading over the entire body if the infant cries hard; veins on the head will swell and throb. You will notice no tears as tear ducts do not function as yet.

Unless your baby is way over the average weight of six to eight pounds, you probably will not be prepared for how really tiny a newborn is. From top to toe measurement may be between eighteen inches and twenty-one inches.

Reach out and touch your baby. Feel that he is warm and slippery. See him move his head and arms and open his eyes. This will be your own little Apgar scoring, one that you will remember your entire life.

NOTES FOR CHAPTER TWENTY-FOUR

1. Arnold Melnick, "The Goal Is a Live, Healthy Baby," *Health* 18: 3–9 (July–August 1973).

2. Rita Kramer, "Revolution in the Delivery Room," *The New York Times Magazine,* July 11, 1976.

Appendix A: Suggested Readings

SEPARATE PUBLICATIONS

Anderson, B. A. *Pregnancy and Family Health.* New York: McGraw-Hill, 1974. (Distributed by the ICEA Supplies Center, P.O. Box 70258, Seattle, WA 98107.)

Auerbach, A. *Parents Learn Through Discussion.* New York: John Wiley, 1967.

Brander, P. *Childbirth Education Instructor's Manual.* Seattle: International Childbirth Education Association, 1969. (Available from the ICEA Supplies Center, P.O. Box 70258, Seattle, WA 98107.)

Bruneau, A., et al. *ICEA Teacher's Guide.* Rev. ed. Seattle: International Childbirth Education Association, 1975. (Available from the ICEA Supplies Center, P.O. Box 70258, Seattle, WA 98107.)

Childbirth Education Association of Rochester, Inc. *Handbook CEA.* Rochester, N.Y.: Childbirth Education Association of Rochester, 1974. (Available from the Childbirth Education Association of Rochester, Inc., Box 9612 Midtown Plaza Post Office, Rochester, NY 14604.)

Clark, A. L. *Leadership Techniques in Expectant Parent Education.* 2d rev. ed. New York: Springer Publishing Co., 1973. (Distributed by the ICEA Supplies Center, P.O. Box 70258, Seattle, WA 98107.)

Cohen, N., et al. *Manual for Setting Up Prepared Childbirth Classes for Cesarean Parents.* Dedham, Mass.: C/SEC, 1976. (Available from C/SEC, 15 Maynard Road, Dedham, MA 02026.)

Consortium on Early Childbearing and Childrearing. *Parenting Curriculum.* Book 1: *Getting to Know Your Baby and Yourself: Prenatal to Birth;* Book 2: *Your New Human: Birth to One Month.* New York: Child Welfare League of America, 1974. (Available from the Child Welfare League of America, Inc., 67 Irving Place, New York, NY 10003.)

Edwards, M. *Communications: Dimensions in Childbirth Education.* Seattle: International Childbirth Education Association, 1976. (Available from ICEA Supplies Center, P.O. Box 70258, Seattle, WA 98107.)

Haire, D., Haire, J. *Implementing Family-Centered Maternity Care with a*

Central Nursery. Seattle: International Childbirth Education Association, 1971. (Contact the authors at 251 Nottingham Way, Hillside, NY 07205.)

International Childbirth Education Association. *Parents and Professionals: Partners in Childbearing.* Convention Report, 6th Biennial Convention, Philadelphia. Seattle: International Childbirth Education Association, 1970. (Available from the ICEA Supplies Center, P.O. Box 70258, Seattle, WA 98107.)

Maternity Center Association. *Guidelines for Teaching: Psychophysical Preparation for Childbearing.* New York: Maternity Center Association, 1963. (Available from the Maternity Center Association, 48 East Ninety-second Street, New York, NY 10028.)

ARTICLES

"Patient Teaching and Counseling." In *Maternity Nursing*, 13th ed., S. R. Reeder et al., pp. 217–35. Philadelphia: J. B. Lippincott, 1976.

Barnes, A. B. Letter: "Prophylaxis in Labor and Delivery." *New England Journal of Medicine*, 294:1235–36 (May 27, 1976).

Bruce, S. J., and Chard, M. A. "Methods of Teaching and Counseling." In *Maternity Nursing Today*, J. P. Clausen et al., pp. 152–68. New York: McGraw-Hill, 1973.

Buxton, C. L. "Psychophysical Preparation for Childbirth." *Clinical Obstetrics and Gynecology*, 6(3):669–84 (September 1963).

Clausen, J. P. "Nursing Leadership of Expectant Parent Discussion Groups." *Journal of Gynecological Nursing*, 2:46–49 (1973).

Goetting, T. "Teaching Resources for Childbirth Educators." *Journal of Gynecological Nursing*, 6:49–55 (May/June 1977).

Hawkins, M. M. "Fitting a Prenatal Education Program into the Crowded Inner City Clinic." *Maternal and Child Nursing*, 1:226–30 (July/August 1976).

Jordan, A. D. Evaluation of a family-centered maternity care program. Part I: "Introduction, Design, and Testing"; Part II: "Ancillary Findings and Parents' Comments"; Part III: "Implications and Recommendations." *Journal of Gynecological Nursing*, 2(1):13–35, 2(2):15–27, 2(3):15–23 (1973).

Miller, H. L. "Education for Childbirth." *Obstetrics and Gynecology*, 17:120–23 (January 1961).

Nunnally, D. M. "A Nurse Establishes Prenatal Program at Med-School Clinic." *Journal of Gynecological Nursing*, 3:41–47 (January/February 1974).

Propper, N. S. "Education for Childbirth in a Rural Mountain Community." *Obstetrics and Gynecology*, 19:563–66 (April 1962).

Roberts, J. E. "Priorities in Prenatal Education." *Journal of Gynecological Nursing*, 5:17–20 (May/June 1976).

Scott, J. R., and Rose, N. B. "Effect of Psychoprophylaxis (Lamaze Preparation) on Labor and Delivery in Primiparas." *New England Journal of Medicine*, 294:1205–07 (May 27, 1976).

Shenk, E. P. "Organization and Conduct of Prenatal Classes and Rooming-In." *Hospital Topics*, March 1963, pp. 90–92.

Stein, T. "Establishing Prenatal Classes in a Small Community." *Journal of Gynecological Nursing*, 2:44–46 (September/October 1973).

Sumner, G. "Giving Expectant Parents the Help They Need: The ABCs of Prenatal Education." *Maternal and Child Nursing*, 1:220–25 (July/August 1976).

Sumner, P. E. "Six Years Experience of Prepared Childbirth in a Home-Like Labor-Delivery Room." *Birth and the Family Journal* 3(2):79–82 (Summer 1976).

Surr, C. W. "Student Nurses Teach Pregnant Teens." *Journal of Gynecological Nursing*, 2:44–48 (March/April 1973).

Thoms, H. "Implementation of a Preparation-for-Parenthood Program." *Obstetrics and Gynecology*, 11:593–95 (1958).

BOOKS

Supplied through the courtesy of:

ACHI Bookstore
Sue Crockett, Proprietor
P.O. Box 1219
Cerritos, CA 90701
(213) 802-1020

Childbirth Education Supply Center
John Crockett, Proprietor
10 Sol Drive
Carmel, NY 10512
(914) 225-7763

CODES USED: qpb–quality paperback
hc–hardcover
pb–mass paperback

A Baby?. . . . Maybe by Elizabeth Whelan. Indianapolis, Indiana: Bobbs Merrill, 1975, $5.95, qpb.

A Baby Is Born by the Maternity Center Association. New York: Grossett & Dunlap, 1964, $6.95, hc.

Anatomy and Physiology of Obstetrics by C. Burnett. Invaluable reference book for midwives and childbirth educators. London: Faber & Faber, 1970, $4.95, qpb.

Birth Book by Raven Lang. Personal descriptions of home births written by a self-taught midwife; exceptional photographs. Felton, Cal.: Genesis Press, 1972, $6.00, qpb.

Birth Goes Home by Lester Hazell. Marble Hill, MO.: NAPSAC, 1978, $3.00, pb.

Birth Primer by Rebecca Parfitt. Philadelphia, Pa.: Running Press, 1977, $4.95, pb.

Birth Without Violence by Frederick Leboyer. Looks at newborn baby as a sensitive and vulnerable human being; encourages a more peaceful birth scene. New York: Knopf, 1975, $8.95, hc.

Cesarean Birth Experience by Bonnie Donovan. A practical, comprehensive, and reassuring guide for parents and professionals preparing for a cesarean birth. New York: Harper & Row, 1977, $8.95, hc, and Boston: Beacon Press, 1978, $4.95, qpb.

Cesarean Childbirth, edited by Barbara Hickernell. Briarcliff Manor, N.Y.: Westchester ASPO, 1977, $3.00, pb.

A Child Is Born by Lennart Nilsson. New York: Delacorte, 1977, $11.95.

Commonsense Childbirth by Lester Hazell. A complete guide for expectant mothers and fathers, giving the natural way. Chapters on home birth and unexpected outcome. New York: Berkley, 1976, $1.95 pb.

Concise Textbook for Midwives by G. Douglas Clyne. Excellent reference material for someone who wants to go into deeper study. Laid out in a question-answer form. London: Faber & Faber, 1975, $9.95, qpb.

Cultural Warping of Childbirth by Doris Haire. Analyzes common obstetrical practices which have distorted the experience of childbirth for parents in the United States. Seattle: ICEA, 1973, $1.00, pb.

Emergency Childbirth by Gregory White. Written especially for emergency birth attendants, but excellent for those planning a home birth. Chicago: Police Training Academy, 1977, $4.00, pb.

Essential Exercises for the Childbearing Year by Elizabeth Noble. Exercises for pregnancy and postpartum revealing role of key muscles—those of the pelvic floor and abdominal wall. Chapter on cesarean restoration, emphasis on prevention. Boston: Houghton Mifflin, 1976, $4.95, qpb.

Experience of Childbirth by Sheila Kitzinger. Stresses importance of harmony of the body with feelings and emotions. Discusses touch relaxation. New York: Taplinger, 1972, $7.50, hc. New York: Penguin Books, 1968, $2.95, qpb.

Faber Pocket Medical Dictionary by P. A. Riley and P. J. Cunningham. Very practical and comprehensive. London: Faber & Faber, 1974, $3.95, pb.

First Nine Months of Life by Geraldine Lux Flanagan. The story of life's beginnings in utero made understandable, fascinating, and beautiful. Authentic and striking illustrations. New York: Simon and Schuster, 1962, $7.95, hc.

From Conception to Birth by Roberts Rugh, *et al.* Detailed and vivid daily diary of embryonic and fetal development. Outstanding color photos of fetus. New York: Harper & Row, 1971, $17.50, hc.

Forced Labor by Nancy Stoller Shaw. The hospital is a factory, the pregnant woman is its raw material. Study describing the routing of women through maternity care systems in the United States. Elmsford, N.Y.: Pergamon, 1975, $5.50, qpb.

Giving Birth at Home by Tonya Brooks and Linda Bennett. Parent information handbook of Association for Childbirth at Home, International. Excellent compilation of all aspects of home childbirth to prepare the expectant couple for their birth. Cerritos, Cal.: ACHI, 1977, $8.00, qpb.

Handbook of Neonatology by Rita Harper and Jing J. Yoon. Functional guide to help recognize emerging neonatal problems. Good reference on the diagnosis and treatment of sick newborns for professionals. Chicago: Year Book Medical, 1974, $9.95, qpb.

Have It Your Way by Vicki Walton. An overview of pregnancy, labor, and postpartum, including alternatives available in the hospital childbirth experience. Seattle: Henry Phillips, 1978, $5.95, qpb.

High-Risk Newborn Infants by L. C. Korones. Textbook for nurses on care of the newborn with chapters on the characteristics, examination, and physiology of the healthy newborn. St. Louis: C. V. Mosby, 1976, $10.95, hc.

Home Birth Book by Charlotte Ward and Fred Ward. Answers most important questions about home delivery. Comprehensive overview covering personal, medical, psychological, sociological, and practical dimensions of home birth. New York: Doubleday, 1977, $5.95, qpb.

How to Relax and Have Your Baby by Edmund Jacobson, M.D. Invaluable help in easing tensions and affording comfort in pregnancy, childbirth, and postpartum period. New York: McGraw-Hill, 1959, $3.95, qpb.

Human Labor and Birth by H. Oxorn. Basic text of normal obstetrics. Englewood Cliffs, N.J.: Appleton-Century-Crofts, 1976, $14.50 qpb.

Husband-Coached Childbirth by Robert Bradley, M.D. Family-centered approach encouraging couples to find their own style in labor. Emphasizes relaxation rather than breathing techniques. New York: Harper & Row, 1974, $8.95, hc.

Immaculate Deception by Suzanne Arms. Compares U.S. childbirth practices with those in other countries. Gives complete information on how hospitals complicate childbirth, presenting a strong argument for home birth. Boston: Houghton Mifflin, 1975, $6.95, qpb. New York: Bantam Books, 1977, $2.50, pb.

Informed Home Birth: A Manual for Parents by Rahima Baldwin. Boulder, Colo: Informed Home Birth, 1977, $5.00, pb.

Is My Baby All Right? by Virginia Apgar and Joan Beck. Prevention, causes, and treatment of birth defects. New York: Simon and Schuster, 1973, $2.25, pb.

Labor and Delivery by Constance A. Bean. Firsthand look at the options available to childbearing women today. Highlights some of the major controversies in obstetrical care as well as alternatives for mothers and fathers who want to take a more active role in determining the quality of childbirth. New York: Doubleday, 1977, $7.95, hc.

Life Before Birth by Ashley Montagu. Influences of the mother to her child before birth. New York: New American Library, 1977, $1.25, pb.

Management of High-Risk Pregnancy and Intensive Care of the Neonate by S. Gorham Babson et al. Conditions that create higher risk to the baby. Prenatal factors that influence the development of abnormalities. St. Louis: C. V. Mosby, 1975, $17.50, hc.

Manual of Newborn Medicine by Gerard Van Leeuwen et al. Typical treatment of abnormalities and disease of newborns in the hospital. Chicago: Year Book Medical, 1973, $9.95 qpb.

Manual of Pediatric Physical Diagnosis by Lewis Barness. Examination of the newborn is covered extensivly. Chicago: Year Book Medical, 1972, $8.95, qpb.

Methods of Childbirth by Constance A. Bean. Overview of different childbirth preparation methods, encourages parents to exercise their options. New York: Doubleday, 1974, $2.50, qpb.

Midwifery by Jean Hallum. Text gives good introduction to basic midwifery. Approaches birth as a normal physiological function. New York: Arco Publishing, 1972, $5.00 qpb.

Midwifery Manual: A Guide for Auxiliary Midwives by Jane Towler and Roy Butler. Chicago: Year Book Medical Publishers, 1974, $16.95, hc.

Midwives and Medical Men by Jean Donnison. Unique history of the development of the midwife and the interprofessional rivalries that exist in regard to women's rights. New York: Schocken Books, 1977, $14.95, hc.

Obstetrics Illustrated by Matthew M. Garrey et al. An informative and easily assimilated text combining general principles with some technical detail, using illustration wherever possible. New York: Longman, 1974, $13.50, qpb.

Pediatrics by Mohsen Ziai. Recommended to parents who want to take an active part in their children's health care from birth on. Also excellent reference for childbirth educators. Boston: Little, Brown, 1975, $15.00, qpb.

The Place of Birth edited by Sheila Kitzinger and John A. Davis. New York: Oxford University Press, 1978.

Practice of Natural Childbirth by Grantly Dick-Read. Abridgment of Dick-Read's writings, a classic of original natural childbirth. New York: Harper & Row, 1972, $1.50, pb.

Pregnancy After 35 by Carole McCauley. Information for expectant parents who are pregnant at an older age. Investigates the various factors involved. New York: E. P. Dutton, 1977, $7.95, hc.

Pregnancy, Childbirth and the Newborn: A Manual for Rural Midwives by Leo Eloisser. Of interest to women in general who want to know what happens and what is done during pregnancy and childbirth. Mexico: Instituto Indigensit, 1976, $5.25, qpb.

Pregnancy, the Psychological Experience by Arthur Colman and Libby Colman. New York: Harper Magazine Press, 1975, $1.95, pb.

Psychology of Childbirth by Aidan Macfarlane. Clear discussion of available evidence of the large number of important psychological unknowns that surround childbirth. Cambridge, Mass.: Harvard University Press, 1977, $2.95, qpb.

Rights of the Pregnant Parent by Valmai Howe-Elkins. How to have an easier, healthier hospital birth—together. How to choose supportive obstetricians and avoid hospital hassles, joining others in the community to effect changes. New York: Two Continents, 1977, $4.95, qpb.

Safe Alternatives in Childbirth by Lee Stewart and David Stewart. Complete transcripts from NAPSAC Conference, May, 1976, plus valuable related information. Chapel Hill, N.C.: NAPSAC, 1977, $5.50, qpb.

A Season to Be Born by Suzanne Arms and John Arms. Beautiful photo essay of pregnancy and birth for the first time. New York: Harper & Row, 1972, $3.50 qpb.

Second Twelve Months of Life by Frank Caplan. New York: Grosset and Dunlap, 1977, $6.95, pb.

Spiritual Midwifery by Ina May Gaskin. Many accounts of home births on a farm commune which are attended by self-taught midwives. Extensively revised and updated with much more medical data. Summertown, Tenn.: Book Publishing Co., 1978, $5.95, qpb.

Teacher's Guide to Manual for Midwives. Mexico: Interamerican, 1976, $1.50, pb.

Twenty-first Century Obstetrics Now, edited by David Stewart and Lee Stewart. Proceedings from the 1977 NAPSAC Conference, with much additional valuable related information. Chapel Hill, N.C.: NAPSAC, 1977, $9.00, qpb.

Why Natural Childbirth? by Deborah Tanzer and Jean L. Block. Demonstrates persuasively why natural methods yield remarkable psychological benefits for every member of the family. New York: Schocken Books, 1976, $3.95, qpb.

Williams Obstetrics, 14th ed. by Louis M. Hellman and Jack A. Pritchard. There is a limited supply of these left. The 15th edition leaves out much valuable information (in the normal sense of obstetrics). Englewood Cliffs, N.J.: Prentice-Hall, 1976, $28.75, hc.

Yoga for New Parents by Ferris Urbanowski. New York: Harper Magazine Press, 1975, $6.95, qpb.

Food and Nutrition

Bake Your Own Bread by Floss Dworkin and Stan Dworkin. Illustrated, step-by-step guide for making and storing bread. New York: New American Library, 1973, $1.50, pb.

Complete Book of High-Protein Baking by Martha Katz. These recipes enable you to enjoy delicious baked goods that are loaded with body-building protein nourishment. New York: Random House, 1975, $1.95, pb.

Cooking with Whole Grains by Mildred Orton. How to cook breads, rolls, cakes, scones, crackers, muffins, and desserts using only stone-ground whole grains. New York: Farrar, Straus & Giroux, 1971, $1.95, pb.

The Dieter's Companion by David Goldbeck and Nikki Goldbeck. Gives a set of principles of food selection that, while allowing great variation in choice of food, enables one to nourish his body wisely. New York: New American Library, 1977, $1.95, pb.

Diet for a Small Planet by Frances Lappe. A plan for eating less meat—or none—and actually improving your overall nutrition. New York: Random House, 1977, $1.95, pb.

Farm Vegetarian Cookbook. To help as many people as possible be vegetarians without turning any of them off or making them think it is strange or weird. To show that a vegetarian diet tastes good, too. Summertown, Tenn.: Book Publishing Co., 1978, $1.95, pb.

Feed Me, I'm Yours by Vicki Lansky. Delicious, nutritious, and fun things you can cook for your kids. New York: Bantam Books, 1974, $1.95, pb.

Grandmother Conspiracy Exposed by Lewis Coffin. Exposing nutritional myths, with suggestions of common-sense ideas for well-fed kids using natural foods. Reveals evils of sugar. New York: Bantam Books, 1976, $1.50, pb.

Let's Cook It Right by Adelle Davis. Easy to follow, tempting recipes, with information on preventing damage done by incorrect cooking methods and harmful ingredients and additives. New York: New American Library, 1970, $2.50, pb.

Let's Eat Right to Keep Fit by Adelle Davis. Tells how proper diet can make you feel better, look younger, and lead a more productive life. Tells what good balances are required and gives diet deficiencies. Points out poisons in additives and manufacturing processes. New York: New American Library, 1970, $2.25, pb.

Let's Get Well by Adelle Davis. How to select the best foods for repairing and rebuilding a sick body. Outlines a nutritional program to aid recuperation and keep you well. New York: New American Library, 1972, $2.25, pb.

Let's Have Healthy Children by Adelle Davis. From the moment of conception, your child's future health and happiness depend on proper nutrition. Complete nutritional guide for expectant mothers, babies, and growing children. New York: New American Library, 1972, $2.25, pb.

Nourishing Your Unborn Child by Phyllis Williams. Excellent information on nutrition in pregnancy. Scores of menus and recipes and cooking methods for natural foods. New York: Avon Books, 1975, $1.75, pb.

Recipes for a Small Planet by Ellen Ewald. Basic and complete cookbook containing hundreds of delicious recipes for better health, better ecology, and better eating. New York: Random House, 1975, $1.95, pb.

Supermarket Handbook by Nikki Goldbeck and David Goldbeck. Guides you past nonnutritive, chemically laden nonfoods in the supermarket to the whole, healthy items still available. Helps to understand labels and select foods with discerning eye. New York: New American Library, 1976, $1.95, pb.

What Every Pregnant Woman Should Know: The Truth About Diet and Drugs in Pregnancy by Gail Brewer and Tom Brewer. Revolutionary book shows women how to safeguard their pregnancies and radically reduce the risks of having birth-defective babies. New York: Random House, 1977, $8.95, hc.

White Paper on Infant Feeding Practices by Center for Science in the Public Interest. Findings and recommendations in line with scientific research and analyses of cultural trends. Washington, D.C.: Center for Science in the Public Interest, 1975, $1.00, pb.

Breast Feeding

Abreast of the Times by Richard Applebaum. Written by a pediatrician, pleads for strong family unit based on love. Miami: Published by the author, 1970, $3.00, pb.

Breast Feeding and Natural Child Spacing: The Ecology of Natural Mothering by Sheila Kippley. Presents a philosophy of mothering; infant's rights to love, care, and the best nutrition. New York: Viking Press, 1977, $2.95, pb.

Nursing Your Baby by Karen Pryor. Comprehensive discussion of how the breasts function and content of human milk. Portrays real adventure of breast feeding in motherhood. New York: Simon and Schuster, 1973, $1.95, pb.

Please Breast Feed Your Baby by Alice Gerard. Historical background of breast feeding. Introduces the idea of breast feeding to mothers who haven't thought much about it. New York: New American Library, 1971, $1.25, pb.

Womanly Art of Breast Feeding by La Leche League International. Practical manual giving information on the how-to of breast feeding—how to overcome difficulties. Emphasizes benefits to baby of good mothering that starts with breast feeding. Franklin Park, Ill.: La Leche League International, 1977, $3.50, qpb.

Parenting

Between Parent and Child by Haim Ginott. Direct, fresh, and easily understood method of communicating with your child, with a relationship of mutual responsibility, love, and respect. New York: Avon Books, 1973, $1.75, pb.

Born to Love by Joann S. Grohman. For women who would like some support for acting and feeling like mothers. How you can restructure natural mothering in your family. Dixfield, Mass.: Coburn Press, 1976, $6.50, qpb.

Distress and Comfort by Judy Dunn. Comforting behavior of parents and its effects on the child. Sensible answers that are useful to both parents and child-care professionals. Cambridge, Mass.: Harvard University Press, 1977, $2.95, qpb.

The Family Bed by Tina Thevenin. Cofamily sleeping to create a closer bond within the family and give children a greater sense of security. Excellent. Minneapolis, Minn.: Published by the author, 1976, $3.95, qpb.

Growth and Development of Mothers by Angela McBride. Exceedingly reassuring for women who are worried about their role and who run into expectations of the "perfect" mother. New York: Harper & Row, 1975, $1.25, pb.

Infants and Mothers by T. Berry Brazelton. Different aspects of normal development of average, quiet, and active babies from birth to one year. New York: Dell, 1972, $5.95, qpb.

Maternal-Infant Bonding by Marshall H. Klaus and John H. Kennell. Impact of the early separation or loss on family development. Importance of early, uninterrupted parent-infant contact. St. Louis: C. V. Mosby, $6.95, 1976, qpb; $8.95, hc.

Mothering by Rudolph Schaffer. Explores the effects of parental care on the intellectual and emotional development of the child. Based on modern studies of interactions between mother and child. Cambridge, Mass.: Harvard University Press, 1977, $2.95, qpb.

Mothering Magazine by Adeline Eavenson. Sharing magazine devoted to information on childbirth, child rearing, parenting, nutrition—all aspects of family life. You may order by single volume—II, III, and

IV—or you may subscribe. Albuquerque, N.M.: Published by the author, 1976, $8.00, one year; $15.00, two years, qpb.

Mother Love by Alice Bricklin. Directed toward people who wish to raise their children in a more natural manner with total family support without some of the modern influences and intrusions. Philadelphia, Pa.: Running Press, 1976, $4.95, qpb.

The Mother Person by Virginia Barber and Merrill M. Skaggs. A candid and serious book designed to prepare women for motherhood as it is in the here and now. New York: Schocken Books, 1977, $3.95, qpb.

Natural Parenthood by Eda J. LeShan. Raising your child without a script, but from your heart. New York: New American Library, 1970, $.95, pb.

Nine Months, One Day, One Year by Jean Marzollo. Goes through pregnancy, birth, and baby care for parents. New York: Harper & Row, 1976, $4.95, qpb.

The Open Home by Sara Stein. Many practical ideas for enriching early childhood. Beautifully illustrated in color. New York: St. Martins Press, 1977, $5.95, qpb.

Rights of Infants by Margaret Ribble. Stresses the vital part mothering plays in the normal development of the child. Good source of the basic needs of the baby. New York: New American Library, 1978, $.95, pb.

The Roots of Love by Helene Arnstein. Shows the indispensable role of love in every phase during the formative years. About feeling of babies, very young children, and their parents. Sensitive guide to hurdles and highlights of unique first love affair between parent and child. New York: Bantam Books, 1977, $1.95, pb.

Your Child's Self-Esteem by Dorothy Briggs. How to help create strong feelings of self-worth. Step-by-step guidelines for raising responsible, productive, happy children. New York: Doubleday, 1970, $2.95, qpb.

Related Subjects

A Cooperative Method of Natural Birth Control by Margaret Nofzinger. Easily understood explanation of a nonsexist form of birth control, requiring love and understanding of both partners. Summertown, Tenn.: Book Publishing Co., 1978, $2.95, qpb.

Free and Female by Barbara Seaman. Explores woman's sexuality in an open and informative manner. Valuable for both men and women. New York: Fawcett World Library, 1977, $1.75, pb.

From Woman to Woman by Lucienne Lanson. Clear, accurate, and sympathetic information enabling every woman to understand the workings of her own body and to discuss any treatment of it intelligently with her own doctor. New York: Random House, 1977, $4.95, qpb.

Helping Ourselves: Families and the Human Network by Mary C. Howell. How families can help each other more and reduce excessive dependence upon the system of managers, experts, and professionals. New York: Harper & Row, 1977, $4.95, qpb.

The Hidden Malpractice by Gene Corea. Massively researched feminist attack on the medical profession and approach to women and female-related diseases. "Knowledge and control of our bodies is the most urgent priority facing women today." New York: William Morrow, 1978, $10.00, hc.

New Handbook of Prescription Drugs by Richard Burack. Essential guide for consumers and professionals to official names, comparative prices, indications for and side effects of hundreds of drugs. New York: Random House, 1975, $1.95, pb.

Our Bodies, Ourselves by the Boston Women's Health Book Collective. Extensive information on the psychological and biological functioning of women. New York: Simon and Schuster, 1976, $4.95, qpb.

Play by Catherine Garvey. How play can be understood as a means of increasing the child's capacity for coping with both physical and social realities. Adds new dimensions to the familiarities of play. Cambridge, Mass.: Harvard University Press, 1977, $2.95, qpb.

Secret of Staying in Love by John Powell. Our greatest gift to one another is a gift of self through the honest sharing of feelings and emotions. Learn a method of communication to accomplish this. For a greater depth in a couple's relationship. Niles, Ill.: Argus Communications, 1974, $2.50, pb.

Touching: The Human Significance of the Skin by Ashley Montagu. How skin is involved physically and behaviorally in the survival of humans. New York: Harper & Row, 1977, $2.95, pb.

Why Am I Afraid to Love? by John Powell. There is a capacity and a yearning to love within all of us that we are afraid to release. We want to give ourselves to others but fear our gift will not be accepted. Niles, Ill.: Argus Communications, 1972, $1.95, pb.

Why Am I Afraid to Tell You Who I Am? by John Powell. Insights on self-awareness, growth, and interpersonal communications. Discusses the human condition, growing as a person, dealing with emotions, and ego defenses. Niles, Ill.: Argus Communications, 1969, $2.25, pb.

The Wisdom of the Body by Walter Cannon. How the human body reacts to disturbance and danger and maintains the stability essential to life. New York: W. W. Norton, 1975, $3.95, qpb.

For Children

Becoming by Eleanor Faison. Focuses on changes a child goes through from conception to birth. Can help children ages three and older appreciate their own magnificence as living beings. Waitsfield, Vt.: Crossroads Press, 1976, $2.95, pb.

Gabriel's Very First Birthday by Sherrie Farrell. Good photographs with text, graphically illustrating Gabriel's birth. Seattle, Wash.: Pacific Pipeline, 1976, $3.95, qpb.

Wind Rose by Crescent Dragonwagon. In exuberant, poetic language, a mother tells her daughter just what she and Daddy felt, dreamed, and planned while waiting for her to be born, as well as the description of the home birth itself. Exquisite drawings illustrate the story. New York: Harper & Row, 1977, $4.95, hc.

Appendix B: Some Sources for Displays, Models, and Charts

American Society for Psychoprophylaxis in Obstetrics
New York City Chapter
P.O. Box 725
New York, NY 10018

Fritz Kallop/Birth Series
Twelve pp., life-size illustrations on labor and delivery, in portfolio case.

J. Bolane
1 San Gabriel Dr.
Rochester, NY 14610
"Fetal Model"—to fit knitted uterus—available in black or white, as a completed model or a sew-it-yourself kit.

Denoyer-Geppert Company
5235 Ravenswood Ave.
Chicago, IL 60640
Sells several models and charts that may be of interest.

Johnson & Johnson
501 George St.
New Brunswick, NJ 08903
"Baby Care Chart" (two-sides: baby care and baby development).

Maternity Center Association
48 E. 92nd St.
New York, NY 10028
"Birth Atlas" (19 charts, 14″ × 20″, bound in an easel-back book; also available as slides).
"Relation of Growing Uterus to Other Organs" (5 charts).
"The Female Pelvis" (1 chart).

"Shape and Structure of Breasts" (1 chart).
"How to Make a Knitted Uterus for Teaching."

Midwest Parentcraft Center
627 Beaver Rd.
Glenview, IL 60025
   "Labor and Delivery Charts" (6 charts, natural color, 20″ × 30″; instructions for mounting).

National Foundation/March of Dimes Supply Division
Box 2000
White Plains, NY 10602
   "Don't Just Count the Months—Make Those 9 Months Count" (counter display with two hinged panels, 27″ × 18″; a multicolor, eye-catching prenatal care exhibit).
   "Light-up Nutrition and Birth Defects Quiz" (2 panels that light up).

Ross Laboratories
Columbus, OH 43216
   "Doll and Pelvis Demonstration Aid" (part of "Prenatal Class Instruction Kit").
   "Nursing Inservice Aid Series" and "Clinical Education Aid Series" (these are appropriate).

Society for Nutritional Education
2140 Shattuck Ave.
Suite 1100
Berkeley, CA 94704
   Great Expectations (16-mm film, color/sound, 23 min. 16 pp. teacher's guide, 30 wall charts, 16″ × 14″.

Trainex Corporation
12601 Industry St.
Garden Grove, CA 92641
   Sells several anatomical replicas that may be useful.

Vitamin Information Bureau
664 N. Michigan Ave.
Chicago, IL 60611
   "Prenatal Nutrition Wall Chart."

Appendix C:
Sources of Audiovisual Aids

CODE: 16 mm — 16-mm movie   c   — Color
S8   — Super 8   b/w— Black and white
S1   — Slide set   s   — Sound
FS   — Filmstrip   min.— Running time (minutes)
AC   — Audiocassette   VT — Videotape
ST   — Sound tape   VC — Videocassette

American College of Obstetricians and Gynecologists
One E. Wacker Dr.
Chicago, IL 60601
   Produces *Educational Materials for Obstetrics and Gynecology* (1974),
      which includes extensive listings for teaching aids, many with reviews.
   The Resource Center will provide information on more recent films.
      Please note that no aids are available through that office.

American College of Obstetricians and Gynecologists Film Service
P.O. Box 299
Wheaton, IL 60187
   Maternity Care Series: 16 mm or VC c s
   Labor and Delivery (1964, 37 min.).
   Medical Examination During Pregnancy (1963, 29 min.).
   Personal Care During Pregnancy (1964, 39 min.).
   Three Faces in Limbo (1965, b/w s 55 min.).

American Hospital Association
840 N. Lake Shore Dr.
Chicago, IL 60611
   Birth by Appointment (1961, 16 mm b/w s 26 min.).
   Hospital Maternity Care: Family Centered (1972, 16 mm c s 25 min.).

American Journal of Nursing Co. Film Library
600 Grand Ave.
Ridgefield, NJ 07657
  Birth Day Through the Eyes of the Mother (1970, 16 mm c s 30 min.).
  The First Two Weeks of Life (1971, 16 mm c s 28 min.).
  Maternity Care: Personal Care During Pregnancy (1964, 16 mm c s 39
    min.).
  Hospital Maternity Care: Family Centered (1972).
  Maternity Care: Medical Examination During Pregnancy (1963, 16 mm
    c s 28 min.).
  Normal Labor and Delivery (1966, VT or VC b/w s 44 min., syllabus
    and guide).
  Preparation of the Breast for Breast Feeding (16 mm c s 10 min.).

American Medical Association Film Library
c/o Association Films
512 Burlington Ave.
La Grange, IL 60525
(Note: AMA Medical Health Film Library catalog)
  Hospital Maternity Care: Family Centered (1972).
  Maternity Care: Labor and Delivery (1964).
  Three Faces in Limbo (1965, 16 mm b/w s 55 min.).
  Modern Obstetrics: Normal Delivery (16 mm c s 27 min.).
  From Generation to Generation (16 mm b/w s 27 min.).
  Maternity Care: Personal Care During Pregnancy (1964, 16 mm c s 39
    min.).
  Age Minus 60 Days (1965, 16 mm c s 16 min [edited]).

American Society for Psychoprophylaxis in Obstetrics
1523 L Street, NW
Washington, DC 20005
  Naissance (1961, 16 mm c s 30 min.).
  The New Generation (1964, 16 mm c s 35 min.).
  The Lamaze Experience (3 33⅓ rpm records, workbook, and chart).
  Labor and Delivery (16 S1 b/w).

Joseph T. Anzalone Foundation
P.O. Box 5206
Santa Cruz, CA 95063
  Becoming (1973, 16 mm c s 30 min.).

A-V Scientific Aids, Inc.
639 N. Fairfax Ave.
Los Angeles, CA 90036

Your New Baby (FS ST).
The Waiting Months (FS ST).
Breast Feeding (FS ST).

BACE (Boston Association for Childbirth Education)
Box 29
Newtonville, MA 02160
A large selection of 16 mm films on the Lamaze method and child care—write for catalog.

Bandera Enterprises
P.O. Box 1107
Studio City, CA 91604
Bathing the Baby (16 mm c s 15 min.).
Age Minus 60 Days (1965, 16 mm c s 20 min.).
The Beginning (16 mm c s 25 min.).

Brigham Young University Media Marketing
W—Stad
Provo, UT 84602
The Miracle of Birth (16 mm c s 30 min.).

Case Western Reserve University
University Circle
Cleveland, OH 44106
Breast Feeding: Prenatal and Postnatal Preparation (16 mm c s 26 min.).

Centre Films
1103 N. El Centro Ave.
Hollywood, CA 90038
The Story of Eric (1971, 16 mm c s 35 min.).

Centron Educational Films
1621 W. Ninth St.
P.O. Box 687
Lawrence, KS 66044
While You're Waiting (1969, 16 mm c s 29 min.).

Childbirth Education Association of Greater Philadelphia
814 Fayette St.
Conshohocken, PA 19428
Birthright (1968, 16 mm c s 15 min.).
Childbirth with Joy (1 33⅓ rpm record, booklet, and 4 leaflets).

Childbirth Education Association of Seattle
7337 27th Ave., NW
Seattle, WA 98107
    Helping Hands (1971, 16 mm c s 36 min.).
    A Story About Childbirth (16 mm b/w s 30 min.).
    Breastfeeding: A Family Experience (16 mm c s 12 min.).

Childbirth Education Films, Inc.
648 Riverside Rd.
North Palm Beach, FL 33408
    First Breath (1971, 16 mm c s 45 min.).

The Claremont Foundation, Inc., Griggs Film Library
P.O. Box 187
Claremont, CA 91711
    Preparation for Childbirth and Two Hospital Deliveries (16 mm c
    silent 35 min.).

Coronet Films
65 E. South Water St.
Chicago, IL 60601
    The Story of Our New Baby (16 mm c s 11 min.).

C.P.E.L. (Childbirth and Parent Education League)
Box 14344
St. Petersburg, FL 33733
    The Joy of Breastfeeding (16 mm c s 15 min.).

Ealing Films
2225 Massachusetts Ave.
Cambridge, MA 02140
    A Child Is Born (1971, 16 mm c s 22 min.).

International Film Bureau, Inc.
322 S. Michigan Ave.
Chicago, IL 60604
    Barnet (The Child) (1969, 16 mm c s 48 min.).
    Pregnancy and Childbirth (1976, 4 16 mm c s 54 min.).

Johnson & Johnson
501 George Street
New Brunswick, NJ 08903
    Baths and Babies (1965, 16 mm c s 17 min.).
    Newborn (1973, 16 mm c s 28 min.).

La Leche League
9616 Minneapolis Ave.
Franklin Park, IL 60131
(Note: Their publication list)
> *Best for Baby . . . Best for You* (1974, 18 min. VC/FS or 56 S1).
> *Mothering Through Breastfeeding* (1971, 16 mm c s 14 min.).

Eli Lilly and Company
Lilly Education Resources
Department M340
Indianapolis, IN 46202
> *After You Go Home* (1969, 16 mm/S8 c s 5 min.).

McGraw-Hill Films
1221 Avenue of the Americas
New York, NY 10020
> *From Generation to Generation* (1960, VT 27 min.).
> *The Child* (3 16 mm c s 85 min.).
> *The First Days of Life* (16 mm c s 16 min.).

Magee-Women's Hospital
Public Relations Department
Pittsburgh, PA 15213
> *A Good Beginning* (16 mm c s 23 min.).

Mead Johnson Company, Inc.
Evansville, IN 47708
> *Hospital Maternity Care: Family Centered* (1972, 16 mm c s 25 min.).
> *Preparation of the Breast for Breastfeeding* (1965, 16 mm b/w or c s
> 10 min.).

Med-Fact, Inc.
P.O. Box 458
Massillon, OH 44646
> Same materials as A-V Scientific Aids.

Media for Childbirth Education
P.O. Box 2092
Castro Valley, CA 94546
> *Birth and Bonding* (30 min S1 AC).

Medical Arts Productions
Box 484

Perennial Education, Inc.
1825 Willow Rd.
Northfield, IL 60093
  A Baby Is Born (16 mm c s 23 min.).
  Birth of a Family (16 mm c s 24 min.).
  Labor of Love: Childbirth Without Violence (1975, 16 mm c s 27 min.).
  Phoebe: The Story of Premarital Pregnancy (1964, 16 mm b/w s 29 min.).
  Unmarried Mothers (1966, 16 mm b/w s 25 min.).

Photoview Instructional Aids
27935 Roble Alto
Los Altos Hills, CA 94022
  Breastfeeding (22 S1 and booklet).
  Infant Care Series (58 S1 and booklet).
  Labor and Delivery, Series I (40 S1 & booklet).
  Labor and Delivery, Series II (44 S1 and booklet).
  Newborn Series (21 S1 and booklet).

Poems & Popcorn
3795 Mission Rd.
San Diego, CA 92109
  American Naissance: Journey with a Friend (1971, 16 mm c s 25 min.).

Polymorph Films
331 Newbury St.
Boston, MA 02115
  Adapting to Parenthood (16 mm c s 18 min.).
  Childbirth (1970, shortened, *Not Me Alone*).
  Gentle Birth (16 mm c s 15 min.).
  Infant Nutrition (16 mm c s 18 min.)
  Not Me Alone (1971, 16 mm c s 30 min.).
  Talking About Breast Feeding (16 mm c s 17 min.).

Proctor and Gamble
Pamper's Professional Service
P.O. Box 171
Cincinnati, OH 45201
  Care for Two: Baby and You (1973, FS, record, 20 min. resource kit).
  The First Two Weeks of Life (1971, 16 mm c s 28 min.).

Professional Research, Inc.
660 S. Bonnie Brae Ave.

Los Angeles, CA 90057
Fairchild cassettes:
  New Obstetric Patient
  Anatomy and Physiology of Pregnancy
  Prenatal Management
  Weight Control and Exercise in Pregnancy
  Course of Labor
  Delivery in the Hospital
  Postpartum
  Breastfeeding
  New Baby Care
  Natural Childbirth

Public Affairs Committee
381 Park Ave.
New York, NY 10016
  Nine Months to Get Ready (1965, 16 mm c s 25 min.).

Rock-a-Bye Baby, Inc.
P.O. Box 24160
Fort Lauderdale, FL 33307
  Rock-a-Bye Baby (LP or tape or AC).

Shelter Books, Inc.
218 E. 19th St.
New York, NY 10003
  The Health Science Video Directory, ed. (1977) by Lawrence Eidelberg,
    270 pp. (note: videotapes and videocassettes only).

Single Concept Films, Inc.
2 Terrain Dr.
Rochester, NY 14618
  Development: 1 Day to 6 Months (1972, VT or VC c s 6 min.).
  The Newborn (1972, VT or VC c s 6 min.).
  Ob/Gyn Series (1973) (VT or VC c s 6 min. each):
  After Your Baby
  False Labor
  Minor Discomforts of Pregnancy
  Preparation for Motherhood
  Questions About Pregnancy

Society for Nutritional Education
2140 Shattuck Ave.
Suite 1110

Berkeley, CA 94704
Great Expectations (1975, 16 mm c s 23 min.; guide & 30 wall charts).

Sterling Educational Films
241 E. 34th St.
New York, NY 10016
Baby's First Four Months (1967, 16 mm c s 18 min.).
The New Baby (1962, 16 mm c s 20 min.).
You and Your Baby Come Home (1966, 16 mm c s 18 min.).
Ladies in Waiting (1966, 16 mm c s 11 min.).
Teenage Pregnancy (1969, c s 18 min.).

Syntex Corporation
Stanford Industrial Park
Palo Alto, CA 94304
A Family Is Born (1970, 16 mm c s 27 min.).

Temple University
Health Sciences Center
Dr. Saul Saltzman
Medical Communications
Philadelphia, PA 19140
Lynn and Smitty (1973, 16 mm c s 17 min.).

Time-Life Films
16 mm Department
43 W. 16th St.
New York, NY 10011
Rock-a-Bye Baby (16 mm c s 28 min.).
Also other related items.

Trainex Corporation
P.O. Box 116
Garden Grove, CA 92642
Infant Care—Breast Feeding (FS, record).
Introduction to Infant Care (FS, record or AC).

University of Illinois Medical Center
Office of Public Information
1737 W. Polk St.
Chicago, IL 60612
Prenatal Care Is for Two (1975, VC c s 28 min.).
When Minutes Count, . . . The Newborn (1976, VC c s 28 min.).
Your Baby and Its Needs (1976, VC c s 29 min.).

University of Kansas Medical Center
Audiovisual Section
Clendening Library
Kansas City, KS 66103
   Proper Care of the Newborn (1971, 16 mm/S8 c s 12 min., 3 parts).

University of Vermont
Dana Medical Library
Audiovisual Department
Burlington, VT 05401
   Birth Day—Through the Eyes of the Mother (1970, 16 mm c s 30 min.).
   Maternal Nutrition (1970, 16 S1).

University of Wisconsin
Bureau of A-V Instruction
P.O. Box 2093
Madison, WI 53701
   Eating for Two (1970, 16 mm c s 22 min.).

U.S. Army Academy of Health Sciences
Attn: HSA-ZMD
Fort Sam Houston, TX 79234
   Breast Feeding (1975, VT or VC c s 13 min.).
   Normal Labor and Delivery (1974, VT or VC c s 11 min.).
   Nutrition in Prenatal Care (1972, VT or VC c s 17 min.).

Vitamin Information Bureau
664 N. Michigan Ave.
Chicago, IL 60611
   Beginning of Life: How a Baby Develops Before Birth (1971, FS script, guide).

Wayne State University
Audio-Visual Utilization Center
5448 Case Ave.
Detroit, MI 48202
   Infant Feeding (16 mm c s 22 min.).

Wyeth Laboratories
P.O. Box 8299
Philadelphia, PA 19101
   Caring for Your New Baby (FS or Sl, AC or records, 4 parts, 52 min. total).

Appendix D: Sources for Childbirth Education Pamphlets

While this list is not exhaustive, it does show the types of organizations that produce and distribute this pamphlet material.

American Academy of Pediatrics
Box P
Post Office Box 1034
Evanston, IL 60204
  Some pamphlets on infant, child, prenatal care, but primarily for the professional.

American College of Obstetricians and Gynecologists
One E. Wacker Dr.
Chicago, IL 60601
  Several items on prenatal care, labor, and delivery—see enclosed catalog.

American Medical Association
535 N. Dearborn
Chicago, IL 60610
  A few items on prenatal and postnatal care.

American Society for Psychoprophylaxis in Obstetrics, Inc.
Suite 105
1523 L Street, NW
Washington, DC 20005
  A variety of items that emphasize the Lamaze method.

Arnar-Stone Laboratories, Inc.
601 E. Kensington Rd.
Mount Prospect, IL 60056
A pamphlet on postnatal postural training.

Ayerst Laboratories
685 Third Ave.
New York, NY 10017
Getting Back Into Shape.

BACE (Boston Association for Childbirth Education)
Box 29
Newtonville, MA 02160
Lamaze method films and books.

Channing L. Bete Co.
45 Federal St.
Greenfield, MA 01301
So You're Going to Have a Baby, 15 pp. 25¢ each.

Blue Cross Association
840 N. Lake Shore Dr.
Chicago, IL 60611
The Modern Baby, 96 pp.

Carnation Company, Medical Dept.
5045 Wilshire Blvd.
Los Angeles, CA 90035
Several items on prenatal and infant care. Note especially: *Pregnancy in Anatomical Illustrations.*

Child Welfare League of America, Inc.
67 Irving Pl.
New York, NY 10003
Parenting Curriculum series.

Cinema Medica, Inc.
664 North Michigan Avenue
Chicago, IL 60611
(312) 664-6170
Distributes a film on home birth, which was supervised by the American College of Home Obstetrics.

Corometrics Medical Systems, Inc.
Wallingford, CT 06492
   Several items on fetal monitoring.

C/SEC, Inc.
15 Maynard Rd.
Dedham, MA 02026
   Materials on cesarean section.

Cutter Medical
Berkeley, CA 94710
   Several items on amniocentesis and ultrasound.

Edcom Systems, Inc.
Princeton, NJ 08540
   The First Years of Life series.

Gerber Products Co.
Box 33
Fremont, MI 49412
   Several items on prenatal and infant care.

Hankscraft Co.
Reedsburg, WI 53959
   The Simple Sanitary Way to Feed Your Baby.

Heinz Baby Foods
Box 28 D-26
Pittsburgh, PA 15230
   Infant and prenatal care; note: *The ABC's of Prenatal Care.*

Hewlett-Packard Company
1501 Page Mill Rd.
Palo Alto, CA 94304
   You, Your Baby, and Obstetrical Monitoring.

International Childbirth Education Association
ICEAS Supplies Center
P.O. Box 70258
Seattle, WA 98107
   ". . . makes available at one center the significant books and pamphlets
   on childbirth preparation, family-centered maternity care, breastfeeding, and related subjects"—ICEA catalog. Offers instructor's kit.

Johnson & Johnson
501 George St.
New Brunswick, NJ 08903
> Several items on infant care, stressing skin care. Note: *Baby Care Course*—student manuals, textbook, instructor's guide, skin-care kit, answer mask.

Kimberly-Clark Corporation
Kotex Products
The Life Cycle Center
Box 551-CK
Neenah, WI 54956
> *Your First Pregnancy* (Vol. VI, the Life Cycle Library).

La Leche League
9616 Minneapolis
Franklin Park, IL 60131
> Several items on breast feeding, including nursing fashions.

Lederle Laboratories
Service to Life Program
Department 785D
Building 140
Pearl River, NY 10965
> Tear-out pages on several subjects.

Maternity Care Association
48 E. 92nd St.
New York, NY 10028
> Several items on childbirth education and maternity care.

Mead Johnson and Co.
2404 Pennsylvania St.
Evansville, IN 47721
> A few items on prenatal and infant care.

The Mennen Company
Professional Service Department
Morristown, NJ 07960
> A few items on infant care, stressing skin care.

National Dairy Council
6300 N. River Rd.
Rosemont, IL 60018

National Foundation/March of Dimes
Box 2000
White Plains, NY 10602
A wide variety of items on prenatal care, maternal and infant nutrition, birth defects, setting up volunteer services; an excellent source for pamphlets.

Ortho Pharmaceutical Corporation
Raritan, NJ 08869
A few items on prenatal and postnatal care.

Patient Counseling Library
Budlong Press Co.
5428 N. Virginia Ave.
Chicago, IL 60625
"A Doctor Discusses" series; offer pregnancy, infant care, and breast feeding.

Pet, Inc.
400 S. 4th St.
St. Louis, MO 63102
Items on formula preparation.

Photoview Instructional Aids
27935 Roble Alto
Los Altos, CA 94022
(415) 948-5832
Distributes 35 mm color slides on childbirth, breast feeding, infant care, and Mensendieck prenatal exercises and movement techniques.

Proctor and Gamble Company
301 E. 6th St.
Cincinnati, OH 45201
"The How to Book on Baby Bathing."

Public Affairs Committee
Public Affairs Pamphlets
381 Park Ave. S.
New York, NY 10016
Pregnancy and You, Nine Months to Get Ready.

The Pyramid Rubber Co.
Ravenna, OH 44266
Modern Methods of Preparing Baby's Formula.

Ross Laboratories
Columbus, OH 43216
> A wide variety of prenatal and infant care materials. An excellent source of information. Note: *Prenatal Class Instruction Kit*: teacher guide, several pamphlets and charts, doll and pelvis demonstration aid, check list, and graduation certificates.

G. D. Searle and Company
Box 1045
Skokie, IL 60076
> *After My Baby—What?*

SIECUS (Sex Information and Educational Council of the United States)
Distributed by:
Behavioral Publications
72 Fifth Ave.
New York, NY 10011
> Series of 14 study guides for sex education. "Sexual Relations During Pregnancy and the Post-Delivery Period" should be noted.

United States Government
Superintendent of Documents
Government Printing Office
Washington, DC 20402
> A wide variety of materials on prenatal and infant care. See especially *Prenatal Care* and *Infant Care*. State and local governments may also provide materials.

Warner-Chilcott
Morris Plains, NJ 07950
> *How to Avoid Constipation.*

Winthrop Laboratories
90 Park Ave.
New York, NY 10016
> Some items on infant care stressing skin care.

Wyeth Laboratories
P.O. Box 8299
Philadelphia, PA 19101
> A few items on infant care.

Appendix E: Schools, Centers, and Clinics for Childbirth Education

Center for Family Growth
555 Highland Avenue
Cotati, CA 94928
(707) 795-5155

People's School of Naturopathic
Health and Institute of the
Healing Arts and College of
Domiciliary Midwifery
928 Fourth Street
Eureka, CA 95501
(707) 442-8717

Discovery Institute
1020 Corporation Way
Suite 103
Palo Alto, CA 94303
(414) 969-3800

Childbirth Without Pain Education
League, Inc.
3940 Eleventh Street
Riverside, CA 92501
(714) 683-9302

Alternative Birth Center
Room 6J5 OB-GYN
San Francisco General Hospital
1001 Potrero Street
San Francisco, CA 94110
(415) 647-7828

Enterpoint Foundation
P.O. Box 88
San Geronimo, CA 94963
(415) 488-9180

Human Lactation Center
666 Sturges Highway
Westport, CT 06880
(203) 259-5995

Home Oriented Maternity Experience (HOME)
511 New York Avenue
Tacoma Park, Washington DC 20012
(301) 585-5832

Maternity Center Associates Ltd.
5411 Cedar Lane #107-B
Bethesda, MD 20014
(301) 530-3300

Birth Day
Box 388
Cambridge, MA 02138
(617) 491-4835

Wholistic Birth and Family Center
P.O. Box 421
Midwood Station
Brooklyn, NY 11230
(212) 693-9230

Healthorium
P.O. Box 59
Lawrence, NY 11559
(212) 471-7308

Centre for Wholistic Birth
934 Washington Street #10
Eugene, OR 97401
(502) 345-3405

Naturopathic Birth Center
671 Southwest Main Street
Winston, OR 97496
(503) 679-6726

Booth Maternity Center
6051 Overbrook Avenue
Philadelphia, PA 19131
(215) 878-7800

The Maternity Center
1119 East San Antonio
El Paso, TX 79901
(915) 533-8142

The National Childbirth Trust
9 Queensborough Terrace
Bayswater, London W23TB
England

Yale University School of Nursing
Nurse-Midwifery
38 South Street
New Haven, CT 06510
(203) 436-3781

Georgetown University School of
Nursing
3700 Reservoir Road, N.W.
Washington, DC 20007
(202) 625-4373

The University of Illinois at the
Medical Center
College of Nursing
Dept. of Maternal-Child
Nursing, Nurse-Midwifery
P.O. Box 6998
Chicago, IL 60680
(312) 996-7800

University of Kentucky
College of Nursing
Albert B. Chandler Medical Center
Lexington, KY 40506
(606) 258-9000

United States Air Force
Nurse-Midwifery Program
Malcolm Grow USAF Medical
Center
Andrews Air Force Base, MD 20331
(301) 981-9811

The Johns Hopkins University
School of Hygiene and Public
Health, Nurse-Midwifery Pro-
gram

615 North Wolfe Street
Baltimore, MD 21205
(301) 955-5000

University of Mississippi
Nurse-Midwifery Program
2500 North State Street
Jackson, MS 39216
(601) 968-5590

St. Louis University
Department of Nursing
Graduate Program in Nurse-Midwifery
1310 South Grand Blvd.
St. Louis, MO 63104
(314) 535-3300

College of Medicine and Dentistry
of New Jersey
School of Allied Health Professions
Nurse-Midwifery Program
100 Bergen Street
Newark, NJ 07102
(201) 456-4300

State University of New York
College of Health Related
Professions
Nurse-Midwifery Program
Box 1216
450 Clarkson Avenue
Brooklyn, NY 11203
(212) 270-1000

Columbia University Graduate Program in Maternity Nursing and
Nurse-Midwifery
Dept. of Nursing, Faculty of Medicine
Columbia-Presbyterian Medical
Center
622 West 168th Street
New York, NY 10032
(212) 280-1754

Simpson Center for Maternal Health
The Community Hospital of Springfield and Clark County
350 South Burnett Road
Springfield, OH 45505
(513) 325-0531

Medical University of
South Carolina
Nurse-Midwifery Program
College of Nursing
80 Barre Street
Charleston, SC 29401
(803) 792-0211

University of Utah
College of Nursing, Graduate
Major in Maternal and Newborn Nursing and Nurse-Midwifery
25 South Medical Drive
Salt Lake City, UT 84112
(801) 531-7728

Index

About the Authors

Dr. Morton Walker, a former practicing doctor of podiatric medicine, ten years ago became a fulltime, freelance medical journalist and author. He contributes frequently to magazines and clinical journals and has published more than 650 articles. He has won eighteen medical journalism awards for research and writing on health subjects, including two Jesse H. Neal Editorial Achievement Awards presented by the American Business Press, Inc., in 1975 and 1976. He has eight published books to his credit.

Dr. Walker is active in the American Society of Journalists and Authors, Inc., which is the professional writers' organization. He was newsletter editor for the American Medical Writers Association, instructor in writing for publication at the University of Connecticut, a newspaper feature writer, a syndicated columnist on nutrition, a radio program producer and commentator over WSTC, and a copywriter for a pharmaceutical advertising agency. From these experiences, Dr. Walker has elected to be a writer of self-help books in the holistic health field. He lives in Stamford, Connecticut, with his wife Joan, and son Jules. Two other sons are married. One is a physician and the other is an accountant.

Bernice Yoffe, R.N., lives in Stamford, Connecticut, with her husband, Sam, and is the mother of two sons, Michael and Frederic. She graduated from the Stamford Hospital School of Nursing in 1941 and served as a Navy nurse during World War II. For the past twenty years she has been employed as an obstetrical and gynecological nurse in physicians' offices.

Nurse Yoffe has been a childbirth educator, lecturer, and Lamaze childbirth instructor for thirteen years. She served on the board of Planned Parenthood of Connecticut and in the Child Guidance Clinic of Greater Stamford, Inc. She is a member of the Nurses Association of the American College of Obstetricians and Gynecologists.

Parke H. Gray, M.D., practices obstetrics and gynecology in the city of Stamford, Connecticut. He graduated from Columbia University College of Physicians and Surgeons in 1962 and did his residency in obstetrics–gynecology at Presbyterian Hospital, New York City.

Dr. Gray has two sons, who were brought into the world by nonparticipating childbirth but who have come out just fine.